I0605624

Eat to Thrive During Menopause

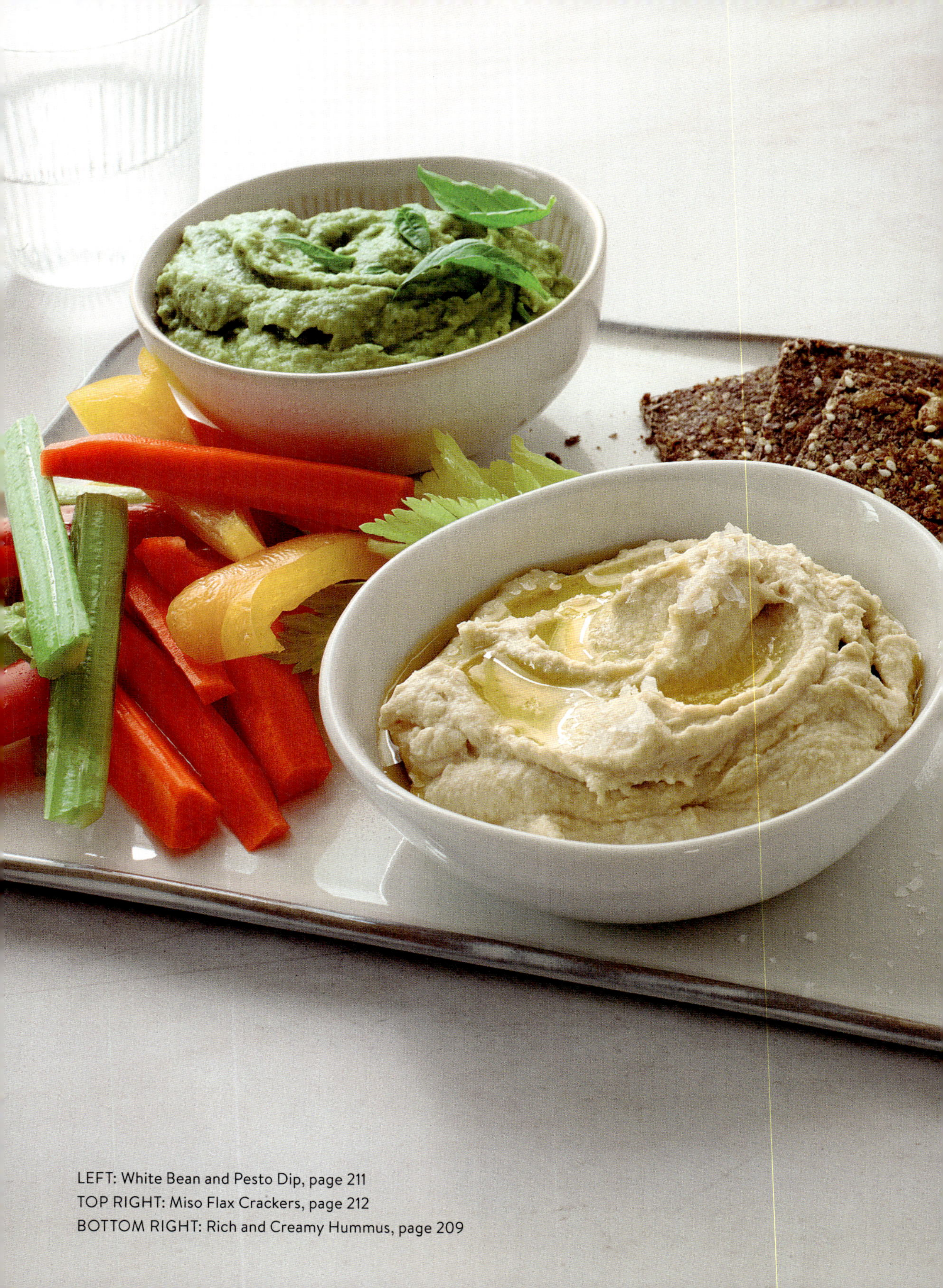

LEFT: White Bean and Pesto Dip, page 211
TOP RIGHT: Miso Flax Crackers, page 212
BOTTOM RIGHT: Rich and Creamy Hummus, page 209

Eat to Thrive During Menopause

MANAGING YOUR SYMPTOMS *with* NOURISHING FOODS

Jenn Salib Huber, RD, ND

WORKMAN PUBLISHING
NEW YORK

Workman
Workman Publishing
Hachette Book Group, Inc.
1290 Avenue of the Americas
New York, NY 10104
workman.com

Design by Becky Terhune
Cover photo by Alexandra Grablewski

Library of Congress Cataloging-in-Publication Data is available.
ISBNs: 978-1-5235-2825-7 (hardcover); 978-1-5235-2829-5 (ebook)

First Edition September 2025

Printed in China on responsibly sourced paper.

10 9 8 7 6 5 4 3 2 1

To my family, who survived my recipe experiments
and still showed up for dinner.

And to every woman who has ever had a hot flash,
may this book make your life a little cooler and a lot more delicious.

Contents

PREFACE

When Early Menopause Crash-Landed into My Life

At thirty-seven, with three children under the age of eight, I blamed my mood swings, broken sleep, and body changes on the stress of having a never-ending to-do list that left little time for self-care. Like most people in their mid-thirties, perimenopause wasn't on my radar, and I was caught off guard when I started waking up at 3 a.m. with night sweats followed by daytime irritability that frayed every last nerve. I also no longer recognized who I saw in the mirror, frustrated by the body changes that appeared seemingly overnight. It took more than a year of visits to various health professionals before I figured out that perimenopause was likely to blame.

I'm happy to say that a lot has changed since then. Menopause is finally getting the attention it deserves—and for good reason. In the United States alone, it's estimated that six thousand women go into menopause every day. By the year 2030, there will be 1.2 billion postmenopausal people worldwide.[1] Thanks to a longer life expectancy, many of us can also expect to spend at least one-third of our lives in postmenopause. If only I'd known in my thirties that up to 20 percent of women will be in perimenopause by age forty and that it lasts four to five years on average—sometimes up to ten![2]

With a diagnosis finally in hand, and nearly fifteen years of experience as a dietitian and naturopathic doctor, I eagerly embraced all the information I could find about how to manage my many symptoms. I also welcomed the opportunity to try hormone therapy, especially to relieve hot flashes, night sweats, and sleep changes. However, after many months of trying various creams and pills, I had to admit that hormone therapy was not right for me. Weighed down by crippling fatigue and low mood from the progesterone (a necessary counterpart to estrogen for anyone with a uterus), my only alternative was to search for nonhormonal support.

As a research enthusiast, I dove headfirst into the world of menopause nutrition. Every book, blog, and guideline offered the same generic advice: Watch your weight, eat more vegetables, and take calcium and vitamin D. I was shocked to discover evidence pointing to many more ways that food can help women manage the symptoms of menopause, especially the most common symptoms of hot flashes and night sweats. Much of this research was published around the same time that we were being told to be afraid of anything hormonal and to fear supposedly estrogenic foods like soy and tofu. And like the evolving understanding of hormone therapy, we can now look back and see that the information we needed was always there, waiting to support a smooth and healthy transition through menopause.

I also realized that this season of life is a crucial window of opportunity to influence not just how long we live but how *well* we live after menopause. For example, during the menopausal transition, bone mineral density decreases by as much as 20 percent and cholesterol levels can increase by up to 15 percent.[3] Simple tweaks to our diets and routines can significantly shift these figures in our favor. What didn't come as a surprise was the need for more credible resources about how to apply this information in an intuitive and practical way that didn't involve cutting out bread or counting, measuring, and tracking every bite of food. It was also around this time that hormone-balancing diets emerged, and the diet-culture grifters wasted no time cashing in.

After more than two decades of experience as a "professional" dieter and teaching others to follow diets and food rules, I learned about the strong case *against* diets. I could no longer ignore the mounting evidence that diets don't work for most people, and I desperately wanted to avoid falling back into the on-again/off-again diet cycle. I was ready to start feeling good about myself and my body—and teach others how to do the same. Around this same time, I was introduced to intuitive eating and the work of dietitians Evelyn Tribole and Elyse Resch, the authors of *Intuitive Eating*. I became a Certified Intuitive Eating Counselor, and this path led me to ways of managing menopause symptoms with gentle nutrition, not rigid food rules. You'll learn about gentle nutrition, one of the ten principles of intuitive eating, throughout this book. It's the sweet spot between what your body wants and needs, and it's exactly what took me from hot, sweaty, and anxious to cool, calm, and collected.

What to Expect from This Book

Eating is instinctual, and yet it can feel impossible to make decisions about food that tastes good, feels good, *and* is good for us. This struggle is exacerbated by the pervasive influence of diet and wellness culture, which distorts our relationship with food, casting a shadow of guilt and confusion over our most basic need. As I often say to women who come to me frustrated because of what they perceive to be a lack of willpower, we have to make decisions about food multiple times a day, every day of our lives, and often with other people's needs in mind. Menopause is difficult enough; what's on your plate shouldn't add to the burden.

My approach unites the science of menopause nutrition with the wisdom of intuitive eating. I can help you redefine your relationship with food, regardless of the stage of midlife you're currently in, so you can thrive, not just survive. I launched my podcast, *The Midlife Feast*, in 2021 because I wanted women to know that menopause doesn't have to be a dreadful experience. Without the distraction of symptoms or obsessing about grams of protein, it can be pretty damn magical. This magic lies in the deepening connection to your own body as you learn to listen and respond to its cues with compassion and understanding. And it's in the newfound confidence that emerges as you embrace this transition with grace, wisdom, and a sense of adventure, knowing that this chapter of life is full of possibilities.

My approach unites the science of menopause nutrition with the wisdom of intuitive eating.

I've spent the past decade helping people navigate the minefield of misinformation about perimenopause and menopause. The women I work with come to me feeling frustrated and lost after trying to navigate midlife and menopause without a road map. They are looking for solutions to help manage what feels like a never-ending list of symptoms. Many are also looking for food peace and are entering this life stage with years of dieting experience in tow. Frustrated by the changing rules of the dieting game, they're ready to welcome a relationship with food that is no longer defined by the scale.

Here I've brought together not only the practical nutritional guidance women need to feel empowered but also a compassionate approach that honors your body's needs during menopause. This cookbook isn't about strict rules, calorie counting, or rigid meal plans; it's about recipes that provide you with freedom and nourishment. My framework will guide you in choosing foods that support your body, energy, and overall well-being, without the stress of measuring or tracking. Instead of wondering if you're "doing it right," you'll learn to trust yourself and enjoy food again, finding ease and confidence in what and how you eat. Together, we'll explore how to feed yourself in a way that feels as good as it tastes—one that sustains your health, honors your changing body, and celebrates this powerful stage of life.

The Four Pillars of Intuitive Nutrition

I have written this book through an intuitive eating and anti-diet lens. The goal is to teach you how to manage menopause without the need to count calories or choose what to eat based solely on its nutritional makeup. The method is based on my four pillars of intuitive nutrition. As you learn to implement the method, you'll appreciate how much easier it is to think of food as a friend, not an enemy.

UNDERSTANDING

Your midlife body needs more than a meal plan. It needs evidence-based advice based on the changing needs of women over forty.

SELF-COMPASSION

You can't hate your body while trying to take care of it. You need compassion, not punishment.

ATTUNEMENT

Intuitive eating teaches you to listen to what your body needs instead of telling it what it should want.

GENTLE NUTRITION

Food matters, but not in the way diet culture has taught you. Let's change your programming around food and health so that eating feels healthy, joyful, and guilt-free!

Before We Begin

Most of this book is written through the lens of the average menopausal experience, with natural menopause occurring around age fifty-one or fifty-two. However, the advice is applicable even if you are in premature, surgical, or medical menopause.

Also, a quick word about the pronouns used in this book: I use "women" and "people" interchangeably to be inclusive of ciswomen and trans and nonbinary individuals experiencing menopause. It is my hope that using both words will make this book feel inclusive for everyone.

INTRODUCTION

The Foundations of a Nourished Menopause

If you've picked up this book, it's probably because you've found yourself in some stage of the transition from perimenopause to postmenopause, and you are looking for a way to include food in how you manage the symptoms you're experiencing. You may have woken up after a restless night of broken, sweaty sleep and wondered if there's something that you're eating (or not eating) that might make a difference. Or maybe the hot flashes you've been experiencing have gone from occasional to nonstop, and you're looking for a way to dial them down a notch. Or perhaps you've watched the women who have come before you suffer their way through midlife, and you want to take action to ensure you're not on the same struggle bus.

You may also relate to the many women I meet who no longer recognize who they see in the mirror and who have spent hours trying to sort through opinions and information about what they should, or shouldn't, eat in midlife. There's a good chance you've even wondered, "Is this menopause or am I going crazy?" Even if you're postmenopausal, you may not feel at home in the "new normal" of this season of life and may feel a bit lost—especially when it seems like every headline is screaming at you about the risks that come with menopause.

You're in the right place if you're interested in learning about how to support your health in perimenopause and menopause with guidance on food and nutrition that's firmly rooted in science, compassion, experience, *and* common sense. I'm so glad you're here.

Setting the Stage for Midlife

Gloria Steinem once said, "The first problem for all of us, men and women, is not to learn, but to unlearn." Anyone who grew up in the 1970s and 1980s watching older women on and off the screen portrayed as dull, boring, and dried up would have a hard time believing that life doesn't end with menopause. Though much has changed, ageism still has far-reaching impacts on women, especially later in life. Many of us hide or downplay our symptoms by saying "It's just my hormones" to avoid inconveniencing others or risk being seen as less competent.

When researchers surveyed nearly eighteen hundred people in midlife and asked about getting older, many described the experience of aging as one filled with shame about their changing bodies, leaving their body image and self-esteem on shaky ground.[1] But there are bright spots, like the Australian research showing that women report being happier in postmenopause when compared to both younger women and even themselves before menopause.[2] And a Danish survey found that women between the ages of sixty-five to seventy-four scored highest on the happiness scale. It's not just those in good health who reported being in good spirits, either. Even those navigating the challenges of an aging body reported being happier than younger counterparts.[3]

It seems that the first thing we need to unlearn is the belief that menopause is an ending. It is *a beginning*, a new chapter. It's time to flip the script.

The Grandmother Hypothesis

History may have prioritized and valued our reproductive roles, but it appears that we, along with a few other mammals, have value far beyond our capacity to reproduce. The grandmother hypothesis suggests that grandmothers' knowledge and resource sharing historically boosted human survival. Similarly, postmenopausal orcas lead their pods, using experience to guide hunts and navigate danger.

In today's world, women over fifty are thriving in new ways—becoming entrepreneurs at record rates, with nearly half of women business owners in the United States now over fifty-five.[4] This vibrant phase of life underscores the value of staying active, strong, and empowered. Hollywood's "past your prime" narrative? Consider it debunked.

The Changing Landscape of Menopause

It wasn't that long ago that the symptoms of menopause, such as mood swings and anxiety, were treated as hysteria, with many women hospitalized or institutionalized during the eighteenth and nineteenth centuries. Even today, depression and anxiety are frequently misdiagnosed and treated only with antidepressants instead of a holistic approach that recognizes these as symptoms of menopause.

Since the early 1990s, research into effective treatments for menopause has grown exponentially, with hormone therapies leading the pack. Following the infamous Women's Health Initiative (WHI) study in 2002, which raised unjustified concerns about the risks of hormone therapy, the use of menopausal hormone replacement therapy around the world dropped by up to 40 to 80 percent.[5] Thankfully, subsequent research and reanalysis of the data from the WHI study have provided a more nuanced and reassuring view of hormone therapy's benefits and risks.

Today, leading experts and reproductive societies around the world recommend hormone therapy as a safe and effective option for most women. Many people credit hormone therapy with saving them from years, or even decades, of suffering. But despite its impressive safety and efficacy, it isn't for everyone, whether by choice or by circumstance. More importantly, it can't act alone, which is why we need an option—one that is accessible to everyone and that can support your body through this transition and beyond, regardless of whether you're using hormone therapy. And that is where the foods you eat come into play, helping you feel better, improve your health, and gain confidence in any stage of menopause. *Eat to Thrive During Menopause* offers simple, science-backed menopause nutrition complete with fifty-five easy, tempting recipes that can start easing your symptoms right away.

How to Undiet Menopause Nutrition

If you google "best diet for menopause" (which I never recommend), you'll end up with more questions than answers. Even as a dietitian with more than two decades of experience, I can still get confused by the volume of information that's out there, so I empathize with anyone who wonders why it's so hard for science and the experts to agree. Simply put, there isn't a one-size-fits-all answer.

I would also argue that we're asking the wrong questions. Instead of asking "What's the best diet for menopause?," which usually assumes that weight loss is the primary goal, we should be asking questions like "How can food help us *feel better* in menopause?" This opens the door to explore the patterns of eating (not individual foods) that can lessen our symptoms and our overall health as we transition from pre- to postmenopause. By asking the correct questions, we can redefine our *why*.

Ask Yourself Different Questions

Instead of focusing on "How can I lose weight?," consider these questions:

1. How do I want to feel?
2. How will my life or health improve if I make changes to what I'm eating?
3. Is there something I'll be able to let go of that will make room for something more meaningful?

These were the goals that one of my clients came up with in response. Some of them might resonate with you, too.

- I want to feel more like myself again and feel confident and comfortable in my body again.
- I want to understand which foods might help manage my symptoms, and hopefully improve my sleep, mood, and energy levels.
- I want to stop second-guessing every bite of food or worrying that I'm doing it wrong all the time so I can free up more space to do things I enjoy.

Undieting is the process of uncomplicating the relationship you have with food so that you no longer let food rules (that are often arbitrary) decide what to eat. It's an opportunity to unravel and build yourself back up with intention. It does not mean you're giving up. Throughout this book, you'll find "Undiet It!" reminders to help you avoid the diet mentality.

The Dos and Don'ts of Goal Setting

It's human nature to want to get things right, ideally the first time. That kind of thinking might work if you're putting flat-pack furniture together, but it's the opposite of how we want to think about food. I used to think that all I needed was a meal plan to make the "right" decisions, a step-by-step how-to guide, complete with lists of "eat this, not that." We've been conditioned to believe that more information is what we need when, in fact, we're drowning in information overload. If you want menopause nutrition to feel easier, you need to do less instead of more. Here are some helpful reminders to keep you out of the dreaded diet mentality:

1. There are no start and finish lines; you're *not* starting a new diet.
2. Food has no morality; it's neither good nor bad.
3. Macros (e.g., proteins, carbs, etc.) aren't magical; all nutrients are valuable.
4. Food isn't only fuel; it's love, culture, and comfort.
5. Food choices should be flexible, allowing for variety and balance.

Build Your Nutrition Capsule Wardrobe

I love busting myths! There's nothing more satisfying than pulling a piece from a precariously built house of cards and watching it fall to the ground. I tackle some of the most common menopause nutrition myths throughout this book—and there's one I want to tackle straightaway because it's the foundation of my method: *Menopause changes everything about our nutrition needs.*

Talk about a good hook, right? If a headline screams, "Watch out! You'd better learn how to eat after forty because menopause changes everything," who wouldn't sit up and listen? Throw in a mention of "meno-belly" and "insulin resistance" and you're sure to find a captive audience. Where's the lie? You're still a human being with a human body, and while it may feel like menopause has changed everything, it has not changed the basics of what your body needs to function and thrive.

How many times have you stood in front of a closet full of clothes and proclaimed, "I need a new wardrobe" when what you actually need is someone to show you how to wear the clothes you have? In other words, you need someone to create a capsule wardrobe with your existing pieces and one or two new items to keep it fresh and in season. A capsule wardrobe is a curated collection of versatile, timeless clothing pieces designed to mix and match easily, which is the approach I take with food and nutrition. In this book, you'll learn how to create a capsule nutrition wardrobe in your kitchen that builds on what you already know about nutrition, then introduces a few key ingredients to help you prepare for anything that comes your way. You'll learn:

- The foundations of building a balanced plate that apply to everyone, regardless of age or menopause stage;
- How intuitive eating can help you declutter the food noise and the food rules that come with it; and
- How to freshen up your daily nutrition with five key ingredients (page 84) to suit your symptoms, individual goals, or health concerns.

In the end, you'll have a plan to include more of the foods you want and need in easy and delicious ways.

Balance Your Plate

It would be unreasonable to expect one type of capsule wardrobe to suit every person on the planet, right? Climate, personal style, and budgets are all factors to consider. However, we can safely assume that most people need a mix of tops, bottoms, underwear, and outerwear. The same is true with food: All bodies need the macronutrients protein, carbohydrates, and fat to function and feel their best. Thankfully, we can be flexible with the foods we choose based on our own tastes and preferences.

In addition to meeting our nutritional needs, the role of pleasure and satisfaction needs to be included in our definition of balance. Just as our clothing choices reflect our individuality and bring us comfort, the foods we select should delight our senses and bring us joy. Savoring a meal that pleases our palate deepens our connection to nourishing ourselves. This is why embracing the pleasure of eating is just as crucial as ensuring we meet our nutrition requirements, creating a balanced and fulfilling approach to food.

Patterns of Eating Are What Matter the Most

Most families cherish a few special recipes passed down through generations that hold a place of honor at birthdays and other celebrations. In my family, it was my nana's peanut butter balls, a Christmas favorite. What makes these recipes endure? Beyond the comfort they bring, they've been perfected over time to turn out exactly right, every single time. The same principle applies to food and nutrition in general. Although new diets and recipes constantly promise to be the healthiest, it's the time-tested patterns of eating that truly promote long-term health, especially during midlife and menopause. I often compare nutrition to a retirement plan—you reap the most benefits from starting early, but it's never too late to make a deposit. When it comes to menopause nutrition, certain key ingredients are on par with your favorite family recipe. But before we dive into those specifics, let's explore a crucial concept: a plant-forward approach.

Setting the Table for More Plants

It's no secret that dietary patterns that prioritize plants are associated with improved health in almost every area, leading some people to wonder if eating *only plants* could be better. While the jury is still out on that question, most experts agree that getting more plants on our plates is a good suggestion. Although vegetarian and vegan diets are nothing new, the recent focus on the benefits of eating more plants has given rise to patterns of eating described as "plant-based" and "plant-forward." As an intuitive eater, I shy away from all-or-nothing labels about food. This is why I've designed this book to be plant-forward instead of exclusively plant-based so that I can equip you with what you need to benefit from more plants, including fruits, vegetables, beans, legumes, nuts, and seeds, without feeling the need to put plants on a pedestal.

How to Make Balance More Intuitive

Imagine you're building a three-legged stool. The seat of the stool is your plate and each of the legs represents one of the macronutrients carbohydrates, fat, and protein. If you try to build the stool with only two legs, it won't be able to stand on its own. Or, if you put two legs close together and the third leg far away, it may be able to stand for only a few seconds. The key is to space the legs in such a way that, even when unequal, they can support the weight of the seat—or plate.

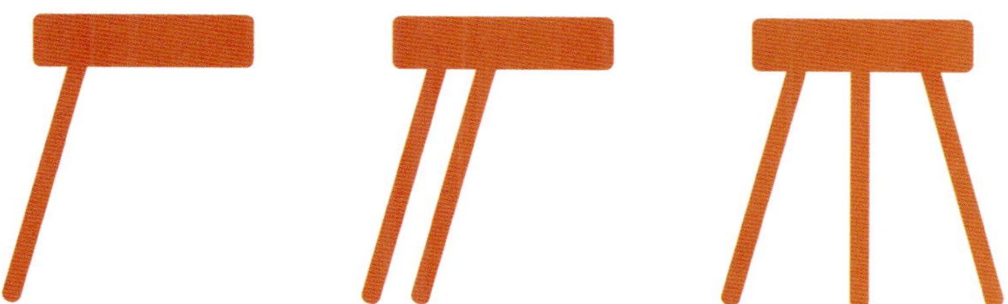

The same is true with food. If you build plates with only protein and fat, the lack of a carbohydrate "leg" is going to leave you feeling tired and irritable because carbohydrates provide glucose, your body's preferred fuel. If you don't have enough fat, your body will have difficulty absorbing the fat-soluble vitamins D and K, necessary for strong bones. Or you may find your meals less filling and satisfying, since fat helps to enhance taste and flavor. Without adequate protein, building and maintaining muscle will be more challenging and satiety will take a hit.

Understanding Macros: Carbohydrates, Fats, and Proteins

The nutrition we get from food comes from two main categories: macronutrients and micronutrients. We get energy from the macronutrients and vitamins and minerals from the micronutrients. Equally essential, they all have a different job in maintaining health throughout our lives, not just in menopause. Despite diet and wellness culture's obsession with protein, or demonizing carbohydrates, learning to view these three macronutrients as teammates who play for the same team, and equally deserving of a place on your plate, will serve you well.

Carbohydrates

Confused about carbs? You're not alone! According to a 2022 survey, seven in ten people believe that the ever-changing landscape of nutrition information makes it hard to know what to believe.[6] Even though most people associate bread, rice, or pasta with carbs, they're also found in fruits, vegetables, beans, and countless other foods. When we eat food containing carbohydrates, they are digested and eventually broken down into glucose, the smallest and simplest of sugars. Glucose can then be used as fuel for cells throughout the body.

Carbohydrates can be classified as "simple" or "complex" based on their structure and how quickly they're digested and absorbed. Simple carbohydrates, such as sucrose, glucose, and fructose, consist of one or two sugar molecules and

Undiet It! The Case for Carbs

Do you have a "less is more" mindset around carbohydrates? Even moderate guidelines for carbohydrate intake recommend getting 40 to 50 percent of total caloric energy intake from carbohydrates, meaning they should still be the dominant macro on your plate. Remember, carbohydrates provide us with our body's preferred fuel. Across almost all cultures, carbohydrates are the fundamental source of energy, provided by foods such as rice, beans, bread, and potatoes. Don't believe anyone who makes the claim that grains are a modern addition to the human diet. There's plenty of evidence that our ancestors have been consuming grains for tens of thousands of years.

provide quick sources of energy. Complex carbohydrates include starches and fibers, which are longer chains of simple sugars that take more time to digest. Starches need to be broken down in the intestine before our body can absorb them, providing a steady, longer-lasting supply of energy. Some examples of complex carbohydrates include potatoes, beans, and whole grains. Fiber, one of the five key ingredients (page 84), is also a complex carbohydrate with a long list of benefits (including the boon of more regular bowels).

Isn't it easier to think of carbs in terms of either fast or slow sources of energy instead of good or bad nutrition? For those of you who've eschewed carbs for fear of weight gain, please know this: The collateral damage of reducing your carbohydrate intake is that you're also removing easy and delicious sources of fiber, vitamins, minerals, and energy—not to mention satisfaction and taste!

Types of Carbohydrates

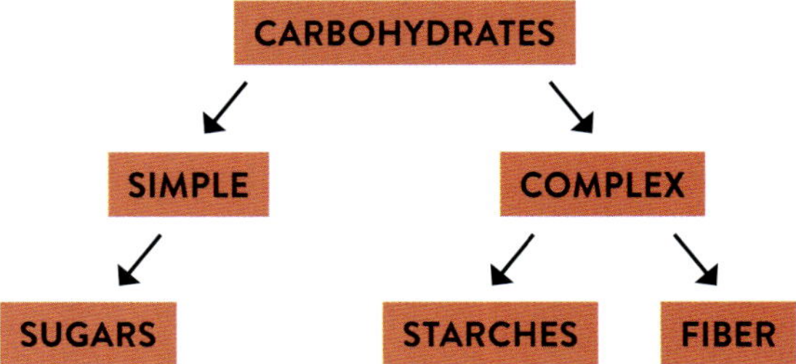

Fats

Like carbohydrates, dietary fats are also divided into two main categories: saturated and unsaturated. Saturated fats are primarily found in foods that come from animals, including meats and dairy products, with coconut oil and palm oil being the only plant exceptions. Unsaturated fats are further divided into mono- and polyunsaturated fats. Another commonality that carbohydrates and fats share is confusion—mixed messages abound regarding what kind is "best" and how much we should eat of any given type. If you're old enough to be in perimenopause, you've probably experienced the extreme "fat is bad" messages of the 1980s, along with the more recent "fat is a superfood" trend that convinced us to put butter in our coffee. So, let's take a moment to undiet what we *think* we know about dietary fat.

We can consider fat in terms of fast and slow energy, just as we did for carbohydrates. Fat is an even denser source of energy than carbohydrates and protein, providing more than twice the energy per gram. Fat is needed to absorb important fat-soluble vitamins, such as vitamins A, D, E, and K. It's also a key ingredient in satisfaction, elevating the experience of eating through mouthfeel and aroma. You only need to think about how much more delicious a piece of warm buttered toast is than a dry one to know exactly what I'm talking about!

The types of fat we eat can influence our health before and after menopause, but the conversation takes center stage when we dive into heart and brain health in particular, as decades of research make one thing clear: There's no need to fear fat, and unsaturated fats should get a front-row seat as their health benefits are well established.

Protein

Unlike carbohydrates and fat, protein has not been subjected to the same scrutiny of its value on our plate. If anything, I would argue that it's enjoyed the benefit of the "if some is good, more is better" mentality, causing many people to feel like they're never eating enough (contrary to the data).[7] Despite protein's unquestionable importance, I would call our cultural obsession with it a sort of "protein mania" that's driven more by marketing than science.

All living things need protein as it's essential for growth and repair. At a basic level, proteins are made up of building blocks called amino acids. Some of these amino acids are considered essential because we can't make them on our own and must get them from food. Sources of protein are typically classified as either animal-based, such as meat, poultry, eggs, and dairy, or plant-based, such as beans, lentils, nuts, seeds, and certain grains.

The discussion around protein, just as with fats, has evolved over time, leaving many of us confused about how much we need and where to get it from. You may remember when the high-protein craze landed in the 1990s and early 2000s, when suddenly it felt like everyone was piling on the meat. And now, with the rise of plant-based eating, there's a renewed interest in getting protein from legumes, tofu, and grains like quinoa. As part of my mission to make menopause nutrition feel easier, let me reassure you that you don't have to devote your life to meeting your protein needs. Although protein is one of our five key ingredients (page 90) and you'll soon learn the types and amounts needed in menopause, for now just remember that protein can't act alone. It needs to be supported by carbohydrates and fats, and it won't be as satisfying otherwise.

Undiet It! Words Matter

Instead of calling a food "healthy" or "unhealthy," talk about its nutrition. For example, instead of saying protein is "good for you," describe it as "filling, satisfying, and important for building muscle."

Eating Is Intuitive

Believe it or not, we're all born intuitive eaters. If you've spent any time with a baby, you know that their hunger and fullness cues are driven not by food rules and schedules but by instinct. Somewhere along the way, we become aware of the expectation to eat in certain ways, that vegetables are good, and too much sugar is bad. These seemingly innocent assertions aren't without harm though, as surveys have found that up to 80 percent of ten-year-old girls have already been on a diet.[8] As you'll learn in the section on body changes in midlife (page 62), the majority of women, many of whom started dieting in elementary school, have spent decades on their quest to find the perfect diet.

Your Mindset Matters More than Your Meal Plan

For the first decade of my career as a dietitian and naturopathic doctor, I lived and breathed the "food is medicine" philosophy. After all, isn't the food we choose the single most important thing we can do to support our health? Although it is true that food can help us in menopause by helping lower cholesterol, cool down our hot flashes, build and maintain strong bones, or keep our brain well fed, we can't ignore our relationship with food either. A healthy relationship with food starts with a healthy mindset that doesn't invite the diet mentality to the table. As we start talking about food and nutrition, I want to help you stay far away from the all-or-nothing thinking that defines many of the books and plans you'll find elsewhere.

The Intuitive Eating Framework

I didn't learn about intuitive eating until my mid-thirties, almost fifteen years into my career. What I love about the approach—developed by dietitians Evelyn Tribole and Elyse Resch more than thirty years ago—is its evidence-based nondiet framework, which can help you build confidence in your eating and nutrition without feeling tied to a set of rules. It teaches you to reconnect with your body's hunger and fullness cues, helps you prioritize satisfaction, and is rooted in body respect and body kindness. It's woven into every aspect of my approach to helping people manage menopause so that finding food freedom and body confidence feels easier than ever.

Intuitive eating has been linked to better health in almost every regard. Studies have found that intuitive eating is associated with improvements in blood cholesterol, blood sugar, and blood pressure.[9] Intuitive eaters are also more likely to choose behaviors linked to better health, such as eating more fruits and vegetables and engaging in physical activity.[10] But one of the most important, in my opinion, is its positive impact on psychological health. A paper published in 2021 compiled the results of ninety-seven studies and looked at the differences between intuitive eaters and nonintuitive eaters. The results made it clear that intuitive eating fosters better relationships with food and our bodies.[11]

The 10 Principles of Intuitive Eating

These ten principles outline the framework of intuitive eating but aren't rules to follow. Think of these as the foundation of a flexible and forgiving relationship with food.

1. Reject the diet mentality: This principle encourages you to let go of the dieting mindset and the pursuit of quick fixes. It rejects the idea that smaller is better or that there's a "best" way to eat. It also calls out the misleading and harmful rules promoted by diet culture.

2. Honor your hunger: Learn to listen to and respect your body's hunger cues and respond by eating when you're hungry, rather than suppressing or ignoring your appetite, which can lead to primal hunger and overeating.

3. Make peace with food: Give yourself unconditional permission to eat all foods without guilt or judgment. This principle helps break the cycle of deprivation that leads to intense cravings, binges, and the feeling that you're losing control. Permission truly is the path to peace with food.

4. Challenge the food police: Challenge and change the critical and negative thoughts about food and eating that often lead to feelings of guilt and shame. These are the thoughts in your head about certain foods being "good" or "bad," which can keep us trapped in the diet cycle.

5. Discover the satisfaction factor: Pleasure from food does not have to be earned. Seek food choices that not only nourish your body but also satisfy your taste buds, promoting a more enjoyable and sustainable way of eating. Satisfaction is the secret sauce!

6. Feel your fullness: Learn to recognize and respond to your body's fullness cues instead of relying on a set of rules or measurements to tell you when to stop. Comfortable fullness is more than simply the absence of hunger; it also relies on feeling satisfied.

7. Cope with your emotions with kindness: Understand the underlying causes of emotional hunger and work to build a toolbox of resources to manage emotional stress, boredom, or other feelings, rather than relying solely on food as a coping mechanism.

8. Respect your body: The world would be boring if we all looked the same. Accept and appreciate that bodies come in all shapes and sizes and that your body is unique. This principle encourages self-compassion and body acceptance, two skills that can improve your overall health.

9. Movement—feel the difference: Instead of moving your body to burn calories, shift the focus of physical activity from weight control to its positive impact on your mood, energy, and overall well-being. Move your body in ways you enjoy and as often as you can and remember that there's no wrong way to engage in joyful movement.

10. Honor your health with gentle nutrition: Food matters but not in the way we've been led to believe. Take nutrition off its pedestal and make food choices that prioritize your long-term well-being while still allowing for flexibility and enjoyment in your eating patterns.[12]

(If you'd like to learn more about intuitive eating, see Resources, page 255).

How to Use This Book

I've written this book in four sections. In part 1, you learn all about the hormone changes you can expect in perimenopause and menopause, and how the different phases of the menopause transition can affect you. In part 2, we take a close look at the most common symptoms of perimenopause and menopause and we discuss heart and bone health. Each symptom has a Kitchen Connection, where I teach you how certain foods and patterns of eating can help you feel more like yourself again.

In part 3, I introduce you to the five key ingredients—soy and phytoestrogens, protein, fiber, calcium, and omega-3 fatty acids. They make menopause nutrition easier by giving you a gentle focus—on adding in rather than taking away—and simplifying the process of deciding what to eat so that it feels more seamless and intuitive. There's no need to count, measure, or track. No complicated rules required. You'll use these ingredients to build a nutrition plan that works for you, regardless of what stage of menopause you're in. Each key ingredient is multipurpose and multifunctional (for example, foods that include protein are usually also good sources of iron, magnesium, and zinc; fiber-rich foods are often high in B vitamins and vitamin E). You'll learn how these key ingredients can reduce symptoms and changes to your health in postmenopause.

Part 4 provides fifty-five simple and delicious recipes that are tagged to highlight their key ingredients, making it easy to select which recipes to make based on your symptoms. For example, if hot flashes and heart health are your priorities, then start by choosing recipes that have the +Soy & Phytoestrogens tag or follow the "Help Me Quickly Hot Flash Meal Plan!" on page 242. You'll find that many of the recipes feature more than one key ingredient, making it easier to add to your nutrition capsule wardrobe.

A Reminder to Choose Integrative Over One Size Fits All

Hormone therapies are, without question, an important piece of the midlife puzzle. Ensuring safe, reliable access to hormone therapy is the priority for most experts around the world, and you won't hear any argument from me. But if declining hormones were the only cause of our symptoms, then hormone therapy would be the cure for every menopause symptom that ails us. There's no question that hormone therapy is effective at treating the most common and bothersome symptoms of menopause, but it's not everyone's magic midlife potion, for any number of reasons.

Menopause is not a *hormone deficiency syndrome* either, the awareness of which some people are advocating for. It is a normal life stage that is also much more than simply a biological event. This is why I believe a bio-psycho-social approach, which considers the factors that influence our health and well-being during menopause, is the best way to support the experience of going through menopause, not only the symptoms. As you're about to learn, my approach to nutrition is a key component of this support system.

As important and powerful as food is, it's not medicine. Likewise, medicine doesn't provide the type of nourishment we get from food. Depending on your personal medical history, family history, and risk factors, hormone therapy may play an important role in how you manage menopause, but it can't work alone. Similarly, hormone therapy will almost certainly cool your hot flashes down, but it won't have much impact on your body composition or body image.

PART 1

Midlife Mayhem

"Menopause is the end of your period, not the end of you."
—Anonymous

Did you know that menopause is actually just one day? It's the day marking twelve months since your last period. The lead-up, called perimenopause, can last up to ten years but typically spans four to five years. Recognizing perimenopause offers a valuable opportunity to influence your experience and set the stage for a life in postmenopause that you'll look forward to instead of fear. The regular and predictable hormone soup you've been making every month since puberty changes as you inch closer to perimenopause, resulting in a medley of physical, mental, and emotional symptoms. Regardless of which symptoms you experience, or when you experience them, they all have one thing in common: Hormone changes are involved.

We All Go Through Menopause

Much like having children, things don't always go according to schedule with menopause. Some women transition naturally while others face a sudden onset due to surgery or illness. Regardless of how or when menopause begins, it is important for women to know that this is a time when self-care and understanding are crucial for overall health and well-being. Understanding the types of menopause—natural, premature, and induced—can help individuals navigate the associated health impacts and treatment options available.

1. Natural menopause: This is when perimenopause and menopause happen spontaneously. The average age for natural menopause is around fifty-one; however, it's considered early menopause if it happens between ages forty and forty-five. Your mother's age at menopause can roughly predict the age when you may go through menopause naturally, but think of it as an educated guess, not a guarantee. Ethnicity, medical history, and even a history of weight cycling in early adulthood can all influence when you go into menopause.

2. Premature menopause: Premature menopause, also called premature ovarian insufficiency (POI), is when menopause occurs before the age of forty. It affects an estimated 1 percent of people with ovaries, and there are some known long-term health

risks associated with it, including osteoporosis and heart disease. Menopausal hormone therapy can help reduce these risks if taken until the expected age of menopause.

3. Induced menopause: Menopause can be induced surgically by the removal of the ovaries (oophorectomy) or can be the result of medical treatments such as chemotherapy or radiation. Both surgical or medical menopause can lead to more intense symptoms and additional health risks due to the abrupt drop in hormone levels.

Our Changing Hormone Soup

Have you ever said "I just don't feel like myself anymore" to a friend or partner? It's so common that researchers have even tried to define what "not feeling like myself" (NFLM) in perimenopause means and found that NFLM was associated with anxiety/vigilance, fatigue/pain, brain fog, sexual symptoms, and volatile mood symptoms.[1] Sound familiar? I lost count of how many times I said to my husband, often through tears, that I just didn't feel like myself anymore.

Throughout most of our reproductive years, we don't give much thought to our menstrual cycle unless it's to avoid pregnancy or become pregnant. As we enter the late reproductive phase, typically in our late thirties or early forties, changes start happening even before hot flashes or missed periods emerge. You might notice heavier periods, irregular cycle lengths, or a decreased tolerance for everyday stressors, like your teenager's messy room. If I could, I'd have a word or two with Mother Nature about the poor planning that has many of us go through perimenopause at the same time our teens hit puberty.

If you're like most women I meet, it might take a while to connect the dots and realize you're in perimenopause. A recent survey found that more than 90 percent of postmenopausal women were never educated about menopause, and more than 60 percent sought information only after symptoms began.[2] Another global survey of seven hundred women revealed that 36 percent didn't understand the difference between perimenopause and menopause, even while experiencing them![3] Can you imagine if we applied these statistics to pregnancy? It would be declared a major public health failure!

The Hormone Roller Coaster of Estrogen and Progesterone

Often described as the "youth hormone," estrogen is the driving force behind your menstrual cycle, playing a role in everything from mood to bone density. Along with its "upstairs hormone" counterparts, follicle-stimulating hormone (FSH) and luteinizing hormone (LH) (which come from the pituitary gland in our brain), estrogen is a reliable ingredient in the hormone soup of our reproductive years, thanks to a well-stocked reserve of follicles in our ovaries.

A quick note about estrogen: Most of the time when you see the term *estrogen* being used, it's referring to estradiol, the dominant form that's most active in our reproductive years. It's also the type used in hormone therapy, and what's measured in a blood test. The other types are estriol, which is produced in pregnancy, and estrone, the main type of estrogen we produce in postmenopause.

As we approach our final menstrual period (FMP), our ovaries begin to sputter, releasing unpredictable numbers of follicles and producing fluctuating levels of estrogen each month. The result is that your roller-coaster ride gets an upgrade, and you may reach new hormonal highs and lows, making your symptoms feel more intense than ever.

Progesterone helps balance the effects of estrogen, and a lack of it can contribute to those crime-scene periods, sleep changes, and even feelings of anxiety and irritability because progesterone stimulates your brain to produce the neurotransmitter gamma-aminobutyric acid (GABA), helping promote calm relaxation. Progesterone may seem like it takes a back seat role, but it's not an insignificant ingredient in the soup. Progesterone rises during the second half of your menstrual cycle, as a by-product of ovulation. Once the follicle releases the egg, it transforms into a progesterone-producing powerhouse. Progesterone levels are first to fall, long before estrogen levels, making progesterone a key player in early perimenopause.

It can be tempting to look at these hormones and try to pin our symptoms on either too much estrogen or not enough progesterone. In reality, it's the fluctuating nature of both key hormones that leads to the symptoms and changes we experience.

What About Testosterone?

Not just for men, testosterone also plays a role in women's health, too, as it contributes to sexual health and libido and may help maintain bone and muscle mass. Testosterone levels peak in our twenties and decline slowly thereafter. By the time we reach menopause, levels are half of what they were at their peak. After menopause, our ovaries continue to make some testosterone even after estrogen production stops. Research into testosterone's therapeutic role in managing menopausal symptoms is ongoing, and I suspect we'll be seeing a lot more about testosterone's role in managing symptoms in the years to come.

Feast on This!

The myth that eating soy foods will lower testosterone levels, or cause men to grow breasts, has been thoroughly studied. The verdict: Neither soy foods nor phytoestrogens (estrogen-like compounds found in plants) have been shown to have any effects on testosterone levels.[4]

Ages and Stages of Midlife: The Menopause Transition

Is this perimenopause or am I going crazy? It's a question I used to ask myself regularly, and one I hear often. There's something about perimenopause that makes everything feel a bit off, like you're living in another dimension. Or more fittingly, another planet. The transition to menopause is a gradual process that doesn't happen overnight, and many people will begin to experience some of the symptoms of perimenopause when they're in what's known as the late reproductive stage, long before they miss a period or have a hot flash.

The Late Reproductive Phase

The late reproductive phase can naturally start as early as your mid-thirties or, more commonly, in your forties. Some researchers use the phrase *very early perimenopause* when describing the late reproductive phase because the symptoms and changes in our experience make it clear that things are winding down.[5] So, even if your cycles are still regular (whatever is normal for you), you may notice some changes, such as:

- Your periods are heavier or more painful.
- Your cycle length is a bit shorter (≤ 25 days).
- Breast tenderness is increasing, especially in the days leading up to a period.
- You're experiencing new mid-sleep waking, what I call the 3 a.m. wake-up call.
- You are hotter and sweatier, especially at night around your period.
- You have new or increased migraine headaches.
- PMS is getting worse and lasting longer.
- Body changes (with or without weight gain) happen despite no changes in exercise or diet.

Early Perimenopause

You might be in early perimenopause if you haven't officially skipped a period but have cycles that are less predictable, coming seven or more days early or late. The roller coaster of hormone changes is in full swing now, and symptoms may appear and disappear from one month to the next, resulting in many people suffering for much longer than needed. A survey of more than one thousand women found that a shocking 68 percent of those in perimenopause did not seek treatment for their symptoms, reiterating the need for education and awareness of perimenopause.[6] In this stage, all of the late reproductive symptoms may still be present (and often more intense), but many people will also start to notice other symptoms as well, such as:

- Hot flashes
- Night sweats
- Body changes
- Skin changes, including acne

Late Perimenopause

In this stage, your cycles will be very irregular, and you may even go months between periods. While these breaks in monthly bleeds can be a welcome relief if you've had heavy and painful periods, the long stretches between cycles may also bring hot flashes, night sweats. and vaginal dryness. Your sleep and mood may still be impacted, and you'll probably notice that your body is starting to go through a redistribution of weight, resulting in your clothes no longer fitting like they used to. (More to come on this on page 30 when we discuss the most common symptoms of perimenopause and menopause.)

Postmenopause

Menopause is the day that marks twelve months since your last period. Many people have a couple of false starts to this countdown, as the timer resets to day one if you have a period anytime in this one-year window (I know, I know). Once you've crossed the twelve-month threshold, you finally enter postmenopause. It might feel anticlimactic—the early years of postmenopause may not feel remarkably different except that you no longer bleed. I often warn people that Mother Nature has a great sense of humor and not to be surprised if you have to reset the countdown in the eleventh hour of the eleventh month. Eventually, you'll get to a point when you feel confident to empty your purses and bags of all the just-in-case tampons and pads you've been carrying around for years. Many women will still experience hot flashes and night sweats during this phase, and some of the other symptoms may have yet to settle down. But many people will feel like they've entered a new normal, with the roller coaster of symptoms finally showing signs of leveling off. It's at this time that the long-term impact of being in a low-estrogen state takes center stage, including the effects on our bones, heart, and brain. This is why having a menopause nutrition plan designed around more than just symptoms is so important!

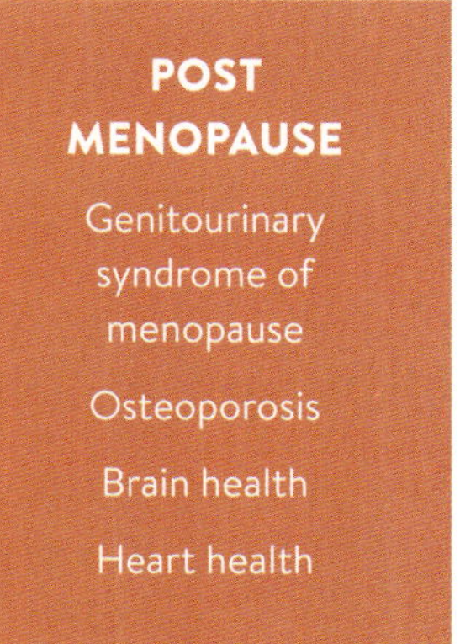

EARLY PERIMENOPAUSE	LATE PERIMENOPAUSE	POST MENOPAUSE
Anxiety	Skipped periods	Genitourinary syndrome of menopause
Mood swings	Hot flashes	Osteoporosis
Body changes	Night sweats	Brain health
Sleep changes	Vaginal dryness	Heart health
Heavier periods	Joint pain	
Cramps	Brain fog	

How Are Perimenopause and Menopause Diagnosed?

Wouldn't it be nice if we had a test that could take the guesswork out of knowing if we're in perimenopause? I would have bought them in bulk a decade ago! Despite the great number of tests on the market that claim to do exactly that, you cannot get a test for perimenopause because it's not something that's diagnosed in a lab.

Your symptoms, medical history, and age, along with changes in your menstrual cycle, are the primary ways to establish perimenopause, not a blood test. What about FSH, the menopause hormone? FSH levels steadily increase the closer you get to your last period, but they can still fluctuate too much to rely on, especially in early perimenopause. I suggest tracking when your period starts and stops, along with any symptoms you're experiencing. This can help you see what stage of the menopause transition you're in now and when you might be moving into another.

I started tracking my cycles when I was thirty-four. By the time I turned forty-one, I was regularly missing periods. Late perimenopause lasted almost three years until my final menstrual period at age forty-four. Like many others in late perimenopause, I spent much of it in the "waiting room" for menopause, often going several months between cycles, each time thinking this was it. I share this with you so that you're not surprised or disappointed if you find yourself having to restart the clock while waiting for menopause to officially arrive.

Is It Perimenopause or PMS?

Premenstrual syndrome (PMS) and perimenopause share many symptoms, making it difficult to distinguish between the two. One early sign of perimenopause that many women notice is a worsening of common PMS symptoms, especially those related to mood, such as anxiety, irritability, and depressed mood. If you regularly suffer from PMS, you might find that your symptoms last several days before your period starts and are more severe than usual.

Another clue is that, unlike PMS, these symptoms may not be limited to the week before your period. You might notice them at various times throughout your cycle. Recent research has shown that people who experience premenstrual disorders like PMS are more likely to go through early menopause and have more severe symptoms. This suggests that PMS and perimenopause have more in common than previously thought.[7]

PART 2

Your Changing Body: What's Happening and What Helps

"I wish someone told me anything, something. All I had heard about were hot flashes. I had night sweats, so I didn't think they were the same thing. I was so uneducated about this phase in my life."
—Gail

Have you ever wondered whether what you're feeling is a hot flash? Or if perimenopause is to blame for your pimples that could give your teenager's acne a run for their money? Or what about the Academy Award–winning mood swing that's gone from a cameo in your life to a recurring role?

As you learned in the previous section, the hormone soup we make in our reproductive years changes once we enter perimenopause. And with those changes come a host of new symptoms. There's no question that menopause would be a lot easier if we had a road map telling us exactly what to expect and when. It makes me both sad and angry that so many women feel uninformed and underprepared for perimenopause and menopause, despite the fact that it's a stage of life everyone with ovaries will go through.

Hot flashes and mood swings are only two of the dozens of symptoms we can experience once perimenopause lands on our doorstep. A quick internet search will yield a list of thirty-four, sixty, or even one hundred symptoms. While thorough, and even validating at times, these lists aren't always helpful because not everyone will experience every symptom, or to the same extent. Tracking your symptoms can be helpful, so I've included a link to various symptom-tracking tools on page 255. It can also be helpful to share your answers with your health care team.

The Study of Women's Health Across the Nation (SWAN) and the Women's Health Initiative (WHI) are two of the biggest studies we have about the symptoms and experiences of people in perimenopause and menopause. This research has helped us understand that even though our experiences won't be the same, some symptoms are much more common than others. According to this research, some of the most common symptoms are:

- Hot flashes
- Night sweats
- Sleep problems
- Mood changes
- Brain fog and cognitive changes
- Body changes and weight gain
- Joint and muscle pain
- Period changes
- Vaginal dryness

In the following section, I describe each of these symptoms in more detail and share the Kitchen Connections that can help you reduce some of these symptoms and prepare for life after menopause. It would be nice if our symptoms followed a set schedule, but unfortunately, that's not the case. More commonly, symptoms come and go, especially in perimenopause when hormone levels are unpredictable. While some are merely a nuisance, others can signal changes to our overall health that shouldn't be ignored.

Hot Flashes, Night Sweats, and Heart Palpitations

Hot flashes take many of us by surprise, even though they're the poster child symptom of menopause. That may be in part because "hot flash" is something of a misnomer—while these symptoms usually involve the perception of heat, they're not necessarily a fleeting zap of white-hot incandescence. Indeed, hot flashes come in various forms, often with heart palpitations riding shotgun. Here's what you might experience:

- Most hot flashes last between thirty seconds and ten minutes, although some can last up to an hour.
- Flushing, redness, and sweating may occur, but not always.
- Even though it can feel like you're about to spontaneously combust in the middle of a hot flash, your core body temperature isn't rising. Thanks to a short circuit in your body's thermostat caused by dropping estrogen levels, your brain gets confused and starts a chain of events to cool you down—cue the hot flash—which results in blood rushing to your skin.
- Palpitations, which feel like a fast or pounding heartbeat, are a vasomotor symptom. Up to 42 percent of perimenopausal women and 54 percent of postmenopausal women report having palpitations.[1] Although palpitations are common during the menopause transition and often don't require treatment, it's always a good idea to bring up any new or worsening palpitations with your doctor.
- Night sweats are hot flashes that happen at night. Some people wake up drenched while others wake up feeling warm and restless.

Hot Flash Contributing Factors

Even though hot flashes are incredibly common, there are other factors that may influence your risk of experiencing these and other vasomotor symptoms.

- **Ethnicity:** Research suggests that Black women are more likely than white women to experience bothersome symptoms, such as hot flashes and night sweats, and for a longer period of time.[2] People of Asian descent report the fewest symptoms.
- **Smoking:** People who smoke (or have smoked in the past) report experiencing more hot flashes.
- **Caffeine:** Coffee and tea can trigger hot flashes in some women.
- **Alcohol:** The frequency and type of alcohol consumed are factors, with red wine often the most problematic.
- **Spicy and hot foods:** Spice, along with the temperature of the food, can impact hot flash frequency.
- **Mental health:** People who experience anxiety and depression may have an increased risk of experiencing hot flashes.

Are hot flashes a universal symptom, experienced around the world? Surprisingly, they might be more common among people living in Western countries for reasons we can't fully explain. Studies show that women in certain countries, including Asian countries, experience markedly fewer vasomotor symptoms. Is it because their diet consists of foods rich in phytoestrogens, including soy foods? Or is it because the culture regarding women's health and experience has not welcomed and provided space for such experiences? More to come on this later.

"Night sweats were my first and most bothersome symptom. I wish I'd known that perimenopause could last well into my fifties." —Melissa

If hot flashes and night sweats are your most common menopausal symptoms, you're not alone—more than 75 percent of women experience them, often beginning in perimenopause, years before missing a period. The as-seen-on-TV portrayal might lead you to believe hot flashes are the same for everyone, but clearly that's not the case. And they arise in four distinct patterns as identified in the SWAN study, each occurring in about 25 percent of the women studied:

1. Early onset of hot flashes, beginning eleven years before the final menstrual period and declining shortly thereafter
2. Later onset of symptoms, with more severe symptoms closer to the final period with a later decline in postmenopause
3. Early onset with a high frequency of symptoms that last long past the final menstrual period
4. Low frequency of symptoms, including no symptoms

The Kitchen Connection

Trust me, you don't need to follow a strict diet or set of food rules to support your health and reduce your symptoms in menopause. Studies have found that including more plant-based protein, soy foods, and fiber and following a Mediterranean pattern of eating can help reduce hot flashes and night sweats.

Soy and Phytoestrogens

It's been almost thirty years since the first clinical trial looking at soy to reduce hot flashes was published in 1995.[3] Since then, at least sixty other studies have looked at the effects of isoflavones, the type of phytoestrogen found in soy foods, on menopause symptoms. Phytoestrogens are plant compounds with mild estrogen-like effects, making them a key focus in menopause research. Even though the results have at times been mixed, several meta-analyses (studies of studies) over the past decade have found an association between soy's isoflavones and hot flashes.[4] Other studies have shown that eating ½ cup (85 g) of soybeans or drinking 1¾ cups (400 ml) of soy milk also makes a significant dent in hot flash severity.[5]

When the research is looked at as a whole, it's clear that there are two important variables to consider with soy's isoflavones: dose and time. A daily dose of 25 to 50 mg of isoflavones, over a minimum of six to twelve weeks, is probably needed before consistent improvements are seen. In my experience, though, people who incorporate phytoestrogen-rich soy foods like tofu, edamame, and soy milk daily can see their hot flashes start to drop in frequency and intensity much sooner, often after just a few weeks. Learn all about this key ingredient in the section on Soy and Phytoestrogens (page 86). You'll also find a "Help Me Quickly Hot Flash Meal Plan!" (page 242) to get you started.

The Mediterranean Diet

The Mediterranean pattern of eating is popular among health researchers, including those who study menopause. A large observational study of more than six thousand people in Australia found that following a Mediterranean diet was associated with a 20 percent reduction in vasomotor symptoms.[6] Similar research has found that eating legumes at least three times a week was associated with fewer and less severe menopausal symptoms.[7]

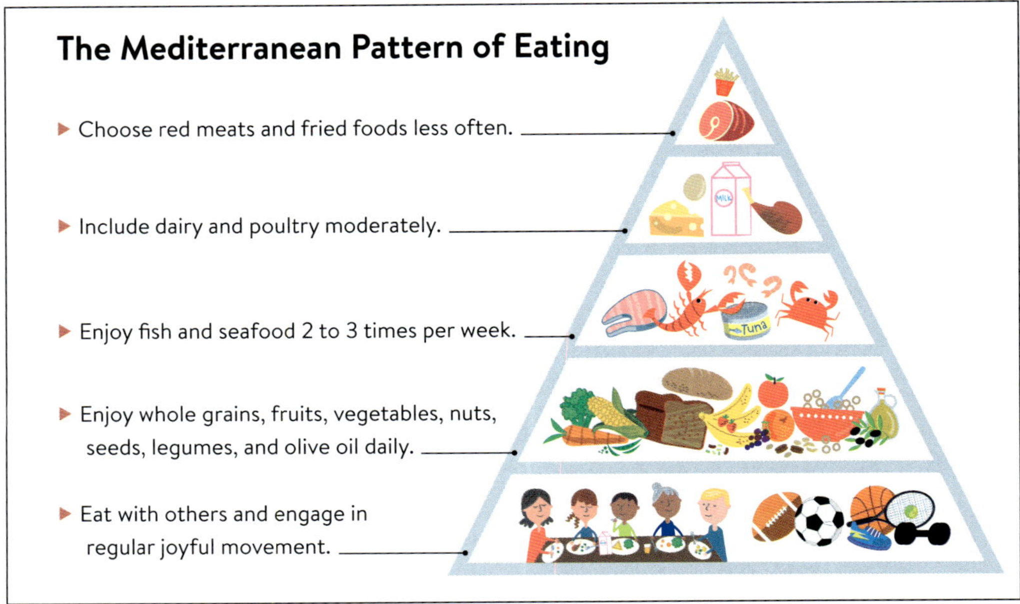

Although the reason behind the Mediterranean diet's cooling effect isn't entirely understood yet, it's possible that phytoestrogens play a role. Even though we tend to associate phytoestrogens with soy foods and Asian diets, phytoestrogen intake from lignans (another type of phytoestrogen you'll learn about on page 88) in some Mediterranean countries has been found to be quite high.[8]

Can You Still Have Coffee and Wine?

Caffeine, alcohol, spicy foods, and even warm beverages are potential hot flash triggers. Try having these less often and see if you notice any changes in hot flash frequency or severity. Try the Golden Soy Latte (page 233) or the Cranberry Mocktail Festive Spritzer (page 237) if you're looking for something to replace an afternoon espresso or evening glass of wine.

On the Menu: Fewer Hot Flashes

If you're trying to eat to beat the heat, you'll want to add recipes that highlight the key ingredient +Soy & Phytoestrogens (page 86) and +Fiber and limit caffeine, especially in the second half of the day.

Breakfast: Tofu Scramble (page 132)

Lunch: Easy Edamame, Dill, and Quinoa Salad (page 199)

Dinner: Mushroom Lentil Stew (page 147)

Snack: Pumpkin Flax Muffins (page 222)

Other Things to Consider

In addition to nutrition and hormone therapy, here are a few other things that may help you manage hot flashes and night sweats.

EXERCISE

- Women who regularly exercise report fewer hot flashes and night sweats. However, some studies have found no relationship between the level of physical activity or exercise and symptoms. It's possible that exercise has an indirect effect on other things such as stress that can't be easily measured. Officially, the Menopause Society, a nonprofit organization whose mission is to promote the health and well-being of women in midlife and menopause, doesn't prescribe exercise for the prevention or treatment of hot flashes, but that doesn't mean it doesn't matter, as it's the best self-care investment you can make![9]

STRESS

- Not to sound like a cliché but try to keep your stress levels in check. Women who report higher stress levels also report having more hot flashes. I once had a patient who suffered with debilitating hot flashes, and even hormone therapy didn't bring much relief. She wrote to me shortly after she retired, pleased to report that her hot flashes completely disappeared once she no longer had to deal with her stressful job.

SUPPLEMENTS

- Studies investigating the possible benefits of supplements on hot flashes have yielded mixed results. Although we can't rule out the possibility that things like omega-3s, vitamin E, or even isoflavone supplements may help, they're difficult to study and research is limited. Popular botanical remedies include red clover, black cohosh, and dong quai. Many women find these helpful, but I recommend working with a licensed health-care practitioner familiar with their use before trying them.

Food for Thought: What Is the Link Between Hot Flashes and Heart Disease?

Although several studies over the past two decades have shown a link between hot flash frequency or severity with an increased risk of heart disease,[10] it's unlikely that hot flashes themselves are the cause. It's more likely that the blood vessel dilation and constriction that occur during a hot flash are related to overall cardiovascular health. Most women experience an increase in heart disease risk after menopause. If you are someone who is experiencing severe hot flashes, now is the perfect time to discuss your family history and other risk factors with your health-care provider. And be sure to keep an eye on cholesterol levels as well, as they can be expected to increase by 10 to 20 percent as you enter menopause.

Sleep Changes

"Will I ever sleep again?" is one of the most frequently asked questions by the over-forty crowd. This isn't a surprise as 40 to 50 percent of women report sleep problems during the transition. As you might know from firsthand experience, it's the difficulty in staying asleep that keeps us up at night, literally!

Not surprisingly, temperature changes (e.g., hot flashes and night sweats) are one of the reasons you might be waking up. One study found that 70 percent of women experiencing night sweats were woken from their sleep.[11] If this is the case with you, it makes sense that treating your vasomotor symptoms should also improve your sleep.[12] People who use hormone therapy that includes progesterone may also benefit from its sleep-inducing qualities.

It's more than just heat that's keeping us up at night as other hormones and neurotransmitters are equally affected by the changing levels of estrogen and progesterone, including cortisol, serotonin, and melatonin. Moreover, people with anxiety and depression may notice that their sleep woes are compounded at this stage of life. The most common sleep changes experienced by women going through the menopause transition are difficulty falling asleep, difficulty staying asleep, and early morning awakenings. And like hot flashes, they can look different for different people:

- New mid-sleep waking (i.e., the 3 a.m. wake-up call) is a common symptom of perimenopause, as are difficulty falling asleep (longer sleep latency) and early morning waking.
- Night sweats and mood changes may exacerbate sleep symptoms.
- People in early perimenopause are more likely to notice sleep symptoms in the week before a period.
- Other conditions such as sleep apnea or restless legs syndrome can exacerbate midlife sleep changes.
- Room temperature, sleep hygiene, and lifestyle factors are contributors as well.

The Kitchen Connection

Is a snack before bedtime a good idea? Should you limit carbs in the evening? The role of nutrition and specific foods on sleep is a growing area of research, and a few themes are emerging.

Food, Hot Flashes, and Sleep

Anything that reduces hot flashes and night sweats (page 31) will probably improve your sleep. For example, Japanese researchers found that over a five-year period, women who reported better sleep quantity and quality had the highest intake of isoflavones from food sources.[13] Similarly, those who eat in line with a Mediterranean pattern of eating may also benefit from better sleep.[14] As we discussed in the section on hot flashes, both isoflavones and the Mediterranean diet may help cool you down.

Food for Thought: What's the Deal with Warm Milk?

A glass of warm milk as a sleep remedy borrows a little bit from science and a little bit from psychology. A warm cup of anything is comforting, especially when prepared by someone who loves us. Milk is a source of tryptophan, along with other amino acids that are known to support sleep. Some studies have also found a link between low calcium intake and sleep, so drinking a glass of milk may help ensure you're getting enough calcium, too.[15] In either case, there's no need to start drinking cow milk if it's not part of your diet already. If you crave something warm before bedtime, soy milk is a source of both tryptophan and calcium, so long as it's been fortified.

The Science of Carbohydrates and Sleep

Carbohydrates bring main-character energy to your sleep. They help shuttle the amino acid tryptophan into our brain, which can then be converted to serotonin and melatonin. And, the type of carbohydrates we eat, along with when they're eaten, also influence overall sleep quality.

Whole grains and complex carbohydrates provide a steady release of glucose into the bloodstream, helping to keep our blood sugar stable day and night. A recent study found that complex carbohydrates, especially those high in fiber, improved somatic symptom scores (which include sleep) on the Menopause Rating Scale.[16] Another suggests that including these fiber-rich carbohydrates may help prevent primary insomnia in menopausal women.[17] I never recommend skimping on carbs, especially with dinner. Research points to an easier time falling asleep if you eat foods containing carbohydrates in the four hours before bedtime.[18]

When considering prosleep dietary tweaks, don't forget to keep it intuitive! Pay attention to how certain foods make you feel, impact your digestion, or influence your sleep. This can help you find the right balance so you don't go to bed feeling overly hungry or uncomfortably full. And women who eat intuitively get an average of twelve more minutes of sleep each night![19] Don't think that sounds impressive? Melatonin, one of the most popular sleep supplements on the market, only nets you an additional ten minutes of sleep.[20]

Sleep and Dietary Tryptophan: A Dreamy Connection

Tryptophan is one of nature's most famous sleep ingredients, responsible for the post-turkey coma most of us have experienced at Thanksgiving. The amino acid tryptophan makes us sleepy because it's a precursor to serotonin, a neurotransmitter that impacts both mood and sleep. Serotonin is also involved in making melatonin, the hormone that regulates our sleep-wake cycle.

After eating foods rich in tryptophan, levels of the amino acid rise in our blood and make their way to our brains. But there's a catch—other amino acids compete to cross the blood-brain barrier, the natural defense system that keeps our brain safe. The secret to getting across? Carbohydrates! Eating carbohydrates triggers the release of insulin, shuttling those competitors into other parts of the body and giving tryptophan a VIP pass into your brain.

Turkey may be the prime example for tryptophan, but it's far from the only good source of this sleep-supporting amino acid. Chicken, eggs, and even soybeans are part of the tryptophan fan club. Including recipes in your diet that feature protein will help ensure you're getting enough. (Research on protein has shown that eating too little or too much may impact sleep quantity and quality.[21] In other words, don't skimp but don't overdo it either.)

On the Menu: Better Sleep

To nourish a good night's sleep, emphasizing foods that are rich in the key ingredients +Soy & Phytoestrogens can help ensure you're getting a good dose of tryptophan and help your hot flashes. It's a good idea to limit caffeine and other stimulants as well, as these can make it harder to fall asleep and stay asleep.

Breakfast: Baked Chocolate Chip Oatmeal (page 121)

Lunch: So Easy Soba Noodle Salad (page 200)

Dinner: Saucy Slow-Cooked Tikka Masala (page 163)

Keeping Your Circadian Rhythm Well Fed

Routine is essential to keeping your circadian rhythm in check. You've probably heard about sleep hygiene, which includes sensible advice about screen time, dark rooms, and not keeping a TV in your bedroom. But have you heard about sleep drive? It is also referred to as sleep pressure, which is the strong urge to get into bed and fall asleep. Nourishing a healthy sleep drive involves good sleep hygiene, but also includes:

- Regular wake and sleep times
- Early morning sunlight (or light exposure)
- Dark room and cool temperature

If it feels like you're doing everything right, but still can't get a good night's sleep, it might be worth looking into cognitive behavioral therapy for insomnia (CBTi), which has been shown to be effective in treating midlife and menopausal sleep woes.[22] You'll find more information in the resources section (page 255).

Meal Timing

Despite what you might have heard, the clock doesn't have much influence on our metabolism, so foods eaten in the evening aren't used as fuel any differently than foods eaten during the day. However, eating too close to bedtime may have a negative impact on how well you sleep. One study found that eating less than an hour before bed was associated with more waking through the night.[23]

Other Things to Consider

There is no quick fix for sleep woes, especially when they're related to our hormones. Keep the following list in mind as you work on getting a better night's sleep.

MOVEMENT

- Research has found that three thirty- to sixty-minute sessions per week of regular exercise, including yoga, walking, fitness Qigong, and aerobic exercise, can improve sleep in perimenopausal women.[24]
- Many of my patients find that vigorous exercise within two to three hours of bedtime can make it more challenging to fall asleep.

SUPPLEMENT:
Magnesium

People in menopause often try magnesium to help with sleep, reduce anxiety, or maintain general health. Although there are many different types you can buy, here are the three most common forms you'll find on store shelves:

- **Magnesium oxide:** The most common and inexpensive form you'll find. It's poorly absorbed, though, so magnesium oxide is most effective for treating constipation and indigestion.
- **Magnesium citrate:** This magnesium is also easy to find and highly soluble, making it popular in powder and liquid forms. It can also help manage constipation and is a good option for people looking to increase their magnesium levels moderately because it is better absorbed than magnesium oxide.
- **Magnesium glycinate:** Magnesium glycinate is the least likely form to have laxative effects and is often recommended for improving sleep, reducing anxiety, and supporting overall muscle and nerve function.

As with any supplement, start slowly and check with your doctor or pharmacist first.

SUPPLEMENTS

- Melatonin is the most studied sleep supplement and may help reduce the amount of time needed to fall asleep but probably won't help you stay asleep. If you decide to try it, keep in mind that less is more when it comes to melatonin, and most studies suggest that doses between 1 and 3 mg, taken one to two hours before bedtime, are most effective.
- Some people find that supplementing with magnesium can help improve sleep. Although research has been mixed on how effective it is, it may help improve sleep duration and quality.[25]

- Studies have found that the herbal medicines ashwagandha, valerian, and passionflower may help with sleep quality and sleep quantity.
- Always discuss supplements with your doctor or pharmacist as many interact with prescription and over-the-counter medications.

Mood Changes

Do the hormone changes of midlife cause mood changes? Or is it that perimenopause and menopause are periods of vulnerability for women who have, or have had, depression? Research suggests that it's a bit of both. Many women experience mood changes such as swings, irritability, and increased susceptibility to depression or anxiety during menopause. The parts of the brain that help regulate mood and emotion are rich with receptors for estrogen, and the levels of the mood-supporting neurotransmitters serotonin, dopamine, and GABA can be taken for the roller-coaster ride.

Many people, including health-care providers, see women in midlife struggling and mistakenly assume that the stress of juggling work, family dynamics, aging parents, and life is to blame. I lost count of how many people dismissed my anxiety as normal because of my hectic life and career. Although it's true that perimenopause and menopause often coincide with busy life stages, this medical gaslighting is yet another barrier for women to overcome. This might explain why a large study of four thousand women found that almost half of women did not approach their general practitioner for help or advice about menopause. Even among those who did, 30 percent experienced delays in diagnosis and treatment.[26] There's no doubt that life can be stressful for legitimate reasons, which makes supporting mental health in midlife even more important. Striking the balance between self-care and caring for others is a challenge many of us can relate to. As with other symptoms, menopausal mood shifts are not one size fits all. Here are some things to keep in mind:

> **"I wish I'd known that meno-rage was not a sign that you are losing your mind." —Trish**

- Perimenopause is a period of increased risk for new or worsening mood symptoms. Women with a history of anxiety or depression may find their symptoms worsen during this transition while others may be experiencing them for the first time.
- Mood changes can range from "not feeling like myself" to full blown anxiety or depression.
- You may experience anger, irritability, and bigger-than-usual reactions to relatively minor triggers. Mood changes in perimenopause appear unique, with less sadness, increased anger and irritability, and greater fluctuation in severity of symptoms.
- Genetics, a previous history of mental health issues, lifestyle factors (such as stress management and physical activity), and social support systems all impact on our capacity to cope.
- Unlike depression, which is often marked by sadness or even apathy, and the tension and irritability familiar to those with anxiety, meno-rage is a unique mix of irritability and white-hot anger that feels like it's erupting from a volcano. The symptom is nearly universal in my experience. And it's often made worse by some of the menopause myths, especially those about avoiding carbohydrates—meno-rage experienced while "hangry" can be an especially volatile combination.

Are hormone changes entirely to blame for all this fun? Or are they simply one of many moving parts that make it feel like we've lost our mind or our filter? Rather than blaming menopause, maybe we have menopause to thank for doing away with that proverbial filter.

The Kitchen Connection

Nutrition is part of the scaffolding of mental health. Mental health, and health in general, improves when our basic nutrition needs are met. And yet, as I've mentioned before, food is still not medicine. People understandably want to know what foods will help them feel less anxious or manage monthly mood swings. I had one woman ask if there was a diet that would help her not yell at her children as often. Of course I didn't have one for her, but I certainly could relate to how she felt. Most discussions about food, nutrition, and mood describe patterns of eating that can reduce the risk of anxiety or depression. There are a few instances where specific nutrients may be noteworthy, but try to keep the idea of scaffolding in mind.

Bank on Balance

Good moods hang in the balance, not the extremes, of nutrition. Carbohydrates and protein work together to make mood-supporting neurotransmitters, such as serotonin, and keep blood sugar and energy levels stable. Fats, especially the omega-3s found in fish and flax, also have a role to play in mood and brain health. Don't leave pleasure and satisfaction off the plate, though, as enjoying your meal will give your mood a boost, too!

Consider the Mediterranean Diet

In 2020, the European Menopause and Andropause Society came out with a position statement on the Mediterranean diet and menopausal health. Among the other benefits of this pattern of eating, it found that it also improved mood and symptoms of depression in menopause.[27] Australia's SMILEs trial found that when people with depression ate a Mediterranean-style diet, they were four times more likely to achieve remission after twelve weeks compared with those who didn't.[28] The foods that are enjoyed as part of the Mediterranean diet are nutrient dense but also delicious, making it easier to want to include more of them!

Other patterns of eating, such as the DASH diet for hypertension, have also been found to improve mood in postmenopausal women.[29] What's important to note is what all of these patterns have in common: They reinforce the importance of eating a variety of nutrient-dense foods, including fruits and vegetables, whole grains, and legumes.

Phytoestrogens and Mood

One of the interesting things about phytoestrogens is that they're able to cross the blood-brain barrier, the very selective filter used to decide what's allowed into our brain. This has led to the suggestion that phytoestrogens, especially the isoflavones found in soy, may have a role to play in supporting both mood and cognitive health.

A logical question to ask is whether soy's potential benefit to mood and depression is related to its ability to reduce hot flashes and night sweats.

Although that is an interesting question, Japanese researchers have found that isoflavones in soybeans improved symptoms of depression in postmenopausal women even when hot flashes weren't affected.[30] We can't yet say for certain that phytoestrogens alone will help, but their potential for having a positive impact on mood is another compelling reason to include them in your diet.

On the Menu: Mood Support

In addition to +Soy & Phytoestrogens, a menu to support improved mood in perimenopause and menopause should welcome foods rich in +Omega-3 fats, including fish, nuts, and seeds.

Breakfast: Toast with nut butter and Very Berry Chia Jam (page 125)

Lunch: Tuna Salad with Cranberry (page 204)

Dinner: Fresh and Crispy Tofu Rice Bowl (page 180)

Snack: Blueberry Lemon Flax Muffins (page 217)

Other Things to Consider

Any plan to support mood in menopause will benefit from an integrative approach. Think of the following important additions to your mental health scaffolding.

INTUITIVE EATING

- Research has found that intuitive eaters report higher self-esteem and overall well-being, along with lower levels of depression and anxiety.[31]

MOVEMENT

- Include a joyful movement practice as exercise has been shown to improve symptoms of depression and anxiety.
- Consider including a mindfulness-based intervention such as meditation or guided imagery to reduce stress and anxiety.

VITAMINS AND SUPPLEMENTS

- Vitamin D deficiency has been associated with depression and anxiety. Your doctor can order a test to check for this, and supplements can help correct a deficiency.
- Although studies are not always conclusive, omega-3 supplements and B vitamin supplements may also be helpful in managing mood changes in menopause.

Period Changes

A changing menstrual cycle is the hallmark sign of perimenopause and menopause. Shorter cycles of less than twenty-five days can be one of the signs of early perimenopause while missed periods signal the arrival of late perimenopause. But the calendar isn't the only place you'll notice a change. You may find yourself dealing with a monthly crime scene, complete with heavy flooding and more cramping than you had as a teenager.

> **"My worst symptom is the very heavy periods. The periods themselves are a problem, but so is everything that comes with low levels of iron." —Leila**

Unsurprisingly, the shift in hormones is usually to blame. If you compare the lining of your uterus to lush green grass, estrogen is the fertilizer that helps it grow while progesterone is the lawn mower that keeps it from growing out of control. It's no surprise then that the unpredictable perimenopausal highs and lows of estrogen and progesterone can turn your monthly cycle into a three-ring circus. Everyone's circus looks a little different. Here's what you might experience:

- Hard-to-predict cycle lengths: They often shorten in early perimenopause and lengthen in late perimenopause.
- Heavy bleeding: If you need to change your tampon, pad, or menstrual cup after less than two hours, or you pass clots the size of a quarter or larger, there's a good chance you're having heavy menstrual bleeding. The official definition of heavy flow is the loss of 80 ml or more of blood during a single menstrual period. That is equivalent to soaking sixteen regular tampons or pads over your entire cycle, as a soaked usual-size tampon or pad holds about 5 ml. If you use a menstrual cup, it may be easier to estimate

how heavy your cycle is, as they usually hold about 30 ml. Heavy menstrual bleeding is common in perimenopause. That said, don't assume that perimenopause is always the cause of your heavy periods (it could be something else, like fibroids); always discuss any new cycle changes with your health-care provider.

- New or increased menstrual pain before and during your period is also common in perimenopause. While often due to fluctuating hormones, it can also be caused by conditions such as fibroids, which are more common during the menopause transition.

The specter of blood-stained pants notwithstanding, the most common side effect of heavy periods is actually iron deficiency, which is already the most common nutrient deficiency among women. It's estimated that one-third of women in the United States (and probably Canada) are iron deficient, with heavy menstrual bleeding being the biggest culprit.[32] The symptoms of iron deficiency include fatigue, brain fog, heart palpitations, and depression—some of the very same symptoms of perimenopause. This overlap makes it difficult for patients and doctors alike to get to the root of the problem. If this sounds like you, have your doctor check your ferritin (the storage form of iron) levels regularly in perimenopause and take steps to ensure it stays within the normal range.

You don't have to be clinically anemic to suffer the effects of having low iron, either. Mild iron deficiency, which happens when your serum ferritin is less than 20 to 35 ug/L, can also result in altered cognitive function, restless legs syndrome, and reduced quality of sleep.[33] In other words, don't ignore heavy bleeding.

Like heavy periods, painful periods are also more common in perimenopause. The fluctuations in estrogen and progesterone can cause the uterine lining to become too thick (or too thin), and conditions such as uterine fibroids or adenomyosis are more likely to develop. Fibroids are benign tumors in the uterus that can cause increased bleeding and pain while adenomyosis involves the growth of endometrial tissue into the muscular wall of the uterus, often causing severe pain and heavy bleeding. (If your doctor suspects either of these, an ultrasound of your uterus can check.)

The pain and cramping are caused by the increase in prostaglandins, a type of hormone that's released by the lining of the uterus. Research suggests that higher estrogen levels and lower progesterone levels are associated with increased levels of these inflammatory hormones, which explains why cramping is more common in perimenopause, when the hormone soup we're making is in flux.

In addition to using anti-inflammatory medications such as ibuprofen, which block prostaglandin synthesis, certain foods and dietary patterns can also play a role in managing pain and inflammation.

On the Menu: Easier Periods

Don't let periods cramp your style. Add foods that feature the key ingredients +Omega-3 and +Calcium while incorporating iron-rich foods on a daily basis. This is especially true if you're in perimenopause and still having regular cycles.

Breakfast: Whipped Cottage Cheese Parfait (page 122)

Lunch: Pea Soup with Feta and Mint (page 140)

Dinner: Cilantro-Lime Chicken Tacos (page 160)

Snack: Choco-Flax Balls (page 216)

The Kitchen Connection

There's no magic recipe or diet that will fix heavy or painful periods. However, when used alongside effective medications and treatments, certain patterns of eating can help smooth the way for a much easier transition.

Eating to Beat Inflammation

Inflammation isn't always a bad thing, and we actually depend on it to mobilize the healing process. But the hormonal fluctuations of perimenopause can result in an overly enthusiastic inflammatory response, which is where certain foods and dietary patterns come in.

Omega-3 fatty acids affect the pathways associated with inflammation and pain. Foods rich in omega-3 fatty acids, including chia seeds, flax, walnuts, salmon, sardines, and edamame, may help support reduced inflammation. Researchers recently looked at the impact of omega-3 fatty acids on period pain and found that diets high in omega-3 fatty acids (including supplements of 300 to 1,800 mg a day) reduced pain and pain medication use in people experiencing painful periods.[34] While more research is needed, the Mediterranean diet, fiber, and even phytoestrogens all show potential in helping to reduce menstrual pain and cramping.

Calcium, Magnesium, and Vitamin D

Calcium and magnesium are involved in muscle contraction and relaxation, and vitamin D plays a role in calcium absorption and prostaglandin synthesis, so it makes sense to consider this trio. Research supports a possible role for these nutrients in managing painful periods, even though most of the research has been done with premenopausal people under the age of thirty.

Several studies have found that as the levels of vitamin D and calcium go down, rates of dysmenorrhea (period pain) go up, and suggest that vitamin D and calcium intake could be effective in reducing the severity of symptoms.[35] Other research has found that calcium supplementation alone (1,000 mg) could be effective in reducing pain intensity when compared to a placebo.[36] Surprisingly, there isn't much research on magnesium for period pain, although many women do find it effective.

Iron

Between the ages of nineteen to fifty, it's recommended that women get 18 mg of iron per day. After age fifty (or more accurately, after menopause), the recommendation drops to 8 mg per day. But it's not as easy as you might think to get 18 mg of iron from food.

Many people assume that if they eat meat, they don't have to worry about iron, but it's not as simple as that. A three-ounce (100 g) serving of beef provides only 3 mg, and chicken even less, coming in around 2 mg. Plant-based sources such as spinach and soybeans look impressive on paper, boasting amounts of 4 to 6 mg per serving, but in reality, they come in much lower because they contain non-heme iron (which the body takes up less readily). However, you can boost the absorption of iron from plant-based foods by pairing them with foods rich in vitamin C.

You might be surprised, but one of my favorite iron-rich foods to recommend is canned oysters! Fresh oysters are great, too, but canned oysters are much more affordable and accessible. A single can provides an impressive 7.5 mg of iron, along with protein and omega-3s. Give them a try.

FOOD SOURCES OF IRON	
FOOD	**Amount of Iron (mg)**
Soybeans, cooked (½ cup/85 g)	4.4
Lima beans, cooked (1 cup/188 g)	4.5
Swiss chard, cooked (1 cup/175 g)	4
Stewed tomatoes, canned (1 cup/255 g)	3.4
White beans, cooked (½ cup/90 g)	3.3
Lentils, cooked (½ cup/95 g)	3.3
Beef (3 ounces/85 g)	2.5
Sardines, canned (3 ounces/85 g)	2.5
Crab (3 ounces/85 g)	2.5
Chicken breast, cooked (3 ounces/85 g)	2
Chicken leg, cooked (3 ounces/85 g)	2

Other Things to Consider

The women I see in my practice suffer much longer than they should with painful and heavy periods. The following suggestions can be game changers if you're dealing with crime-scene periods.

MEDICATIONS AND SUPPLEMENTS

- Talk to your doctor about using progesterone to help manage your heavy periods. Both the oral form of progesterone and progestin IUDs can significantly reduce heavy menstrual bleeding. There are also nonhormonal medication options available.
- Vitamin D supplements show promise in reducing menstrual pain in younger women, but research is lacking for women in perimenopause.[37]

MOVEMENT

- Regular movement, including yoga, walking, and other types of exercise, can reduce pain and cramping.[38]

Muscle and Joint Pain

More than 50 percent of women who are going through perimenopause and menopause will experience some kind of muscle and joint pain. You might notice that you're stiffer when you get out of bed in the morning or that standing up after a long period of sitting isn't quite as easy as it used to be. Is it osteoarthritis? Is this simply a function of getting older? Somewhat, as both men and women experience these symptoms. But there's more going on than just aging, and it seems likely that menopause is involved.

The effect of estrogen loss on muscle and joint pain isn't completely understood, but we do know that estrogen influences both inflammation and repair and that connective tissue, like the cartilage that cushions our joints, has receptors for estrogen. This fact, along with age-related changes to the natural joint lubrication that keeps things moving, might explain why the rates of soft tissue injuries, including tendonitis and frozen shoulder, increase in perimenopause and menopause.

> **"I was surprised by the *amount* of back and hip pain I developed. I wasn't prepared for how much it would affect my mental state."**
> **—Cory**

Estrogen isn't the whole story, though. Equally important are the connections among age, estrogen, and muscle. We know that it gets harder to build and maintain muscle as we age. Between the ages of thirty and sixty, the average adult loses about 3 to 5 percent of muscle per decade.[39] This accelerates during perimenopause before leveling off again in postmenopause, but it's possible to slow it down by moving your body regularly, including strength training, and eating in a way that helps your body build and maintain muscle. (For more on this, see page 91.)

Just like adolescent growing pains, menopausal body aches can look different for each of us. Here's what you might experience:

- Musculoskeletal pain can affect muscles, ligaments, tendons, and bones. The pain can be short-lived or persist for many months, or even years. Sometimes the pain feels like it's in a specific place or places; other times, it can abate in one area and surface in another. As some patients report—particularly at the end of a long day—it's the sensation of "everything hurts."

- Many women will experience joint stiffness and pain (arthralgia), muscle aches, or bone pain during perimenopause, and rates of osteoarthritis increase over the transition.
- Many women find that their joint and muscle pain improves with hormone therapy, but others don't. This is why experts don't recommend hormone therapy as first-line therapy for menopause-associated joint pain, but it may be a side benefit.

The Kitchen Connection

How we nourish ourselves has the potential to influence pain and inflammation, but no single food or food group is to blame for our midlife aches and stiffness. Although certain nutrients including vitamin D, omega-3 fatty acids, magnesium, and even isoflavones are noteworthy, you should be skeptical about any food or meal plan that promises to cure pain of any kind.

Anti-Inflammatory Diets

Inflammation is high on the list of trendy buzzwords, and diet culture wasted no time jumping on board, blaming everything from high-sugar diets to lectins found in everyday foods like grains and lentils. Although inflammation can certainly cause pain in some instances, it's important to remember that not all pain is the result of inflammation, and not all inflammation is problematic.

Acute inflammation is an inherently healing response to injury or infection, such as a cut or scrape. In these cases, we don't want to stop or slow it down, as it's an essential part of the process. Chronic inflammation is different and is emerging as a potential risk factor for everything from diabetes to dementia. Understanding what role food can play in reducing chronic inflammation is worthy of consideration, but keep in mind that research linking specific foods to chronic inflammation is sparse and that the strongest recommendations are made for patterns of eating, not specific foods or nutrients.

Considering your patterns of eating may be helpful. One study, which looked at the effect of dietary patterns on inflammatory markers that can be measured in our blood, found that many of the well-known health-promoting eating patterns (such as the Mediterranean diet) could significantly reduce levels of the inflammatory marker called C-reactive protein, or CRP.[40] Although the Mediterranean diet's impact on menopausal joint pain has not been looked at specifically, several studies have found links between it and reduced pain in other conditions, including osteoarthritis and rheumatoid arthritis. So, it's reasonable to assume that this pattern of eating may help decrease pain and inflammation.

These patterns also recommend consuming fish (preferably oily fish) at least once a week. Omega-3s, especially those from fish, are among the most popular supplements for joint pain, and many women find them helpful even though the evidence is limited.

Undiet It! The Truth About Sugar and Inflammation

Are sugar-laden foods responsible for inflammation and our aches and pains? Most of the evidence suggesting a link between sugar and inflammation comes from observational studies of sugar-sweetened beverages. These types of studies can only establish correlation, not causation, between two things. Results from human trials largely have been inconclusive, with most pointing to the pattern of eating (not sugar specifically) as the link between food and inflammation.

Dial in Diversity

Dietary diversity refers to the variety or the number of different *food groups* (not individual foods) consumed over a given period, and eating with dietary diversity in mind can help ensure adequate nutrient intake and promote overall health. A study examining dietary diversity and musculoskeletal pain found that older adults who maintained a more diverse diet experienced less joint pain.[41] Another reason to embrace intuitive eating and welcome all foods to the table—variety for the win!

On the Menu: Healthy Joints and Muscles

An important feature of supporting musculoskeletal health in midlife is keeping our muscles strong and healthy. For this reason, the key ingredient +Protein deserves a spot on your menu alongside +Soy & Phytoestrogens and +Omega-3 for anti-inflammatory support.

Breakfast: Carrot Cake Overnight Oats (page 117)

Lunch: Smashed Chickpea Salad (page 195)

Dinner: Sheet-Pan Pistachio-Crusted Fish and Roasted Potatoes (page 174)

Snack: Chia Seed Pudding (page 225)

Soy and Phytoestrogens

Soy is somewhat unique in that it's one of the few complete plant-based proteins, meaning it contains all of the essential amino acids needed for growth and repair. Researchers studying soy's possible role in reducing inflammation suggest that soy foods may also lower the inflammatory CRP marker.[42] Soy protein also outperformed whey protein in a study that looked at various inflammatory markers, noting that isoflavones, the type of phystoestrogens found in soy foods, may be responsible for this.[43]

Protein

As we get older our body may not use protein as efficiently as it used to in building and maintaining muscle. This is the reason behind the "eat more protein" message you've probably seen or heard. Although it's true that protein needs increase slightly as we age, I want to reassure you that you don't need to devote your life to eating protein, as some influencers would like you to believe. As you'll learn on page 94, there are many delicious and satisfying ways to include adequate amounts of protein to build and maintain muscle and strength.

Turmeric

Turmeric is a bright yellow spice that has become popular for its antioxidant and anti-inflammatory effects. Many are surprised to hear that, despite its delicious flavor and bright color, its use in the kitchen probably *won't* help your aches and pains. Turmeric contains only about 2 to 6 percent curcumin, the active ingredient that's linked to reduced inflammation and pain. It is delicious, though, so give the Golden Soy Latte (page 233) a try.

Other Things to Consider

Keep the following in mind if you feel like you need an all-hands-on-deck approach to midlife muscle and joint pain:

MOVEMENT

- Up your strength game: Research has found that strength and resistance training can reduce pain and improve function in people with knee osteoarthritis.[44]

SUPPLEMENTS

- Although evidence is mixed for glucosamine, chondroitin, and magnesium, many women find these supplements helpful.
- Hydrolyzed collagen supplements are popular, but the jury is still out on their effectiveness for joint pain. If you do decide to try them, research suggests taking 10 to 20 g per day for a minimum of six to eight weeks.

Feast on This!

Do foods from the nightshade family, such as tomatoes, potatoes, and peppers, worsen joint pain and arthritis? Probably not. Foods from the nightshade family contain solanine, an alkaloid that can be toxic and pro-inflammatory in large amounts. But it's most concentrated in the leaves and stems of the plants, not the parts we eat. Research does not support the idea that foods from the nightshade family have a negative effect on joint pain or make arthritis worse.

Cognitive Health

Most of our menopause symptoms start in the brain, not the ovaries. Even hot flashes are the result of a malfunctioning thermostat (page 31). And because our brains are richly populated with hormone receptors and hardwired to run on estrogen, the fluctuating hormone soup of perimenopause can be especially uncomfortable to say the least.

Have you ever turned down the volume on the car radio to see better while driving? I'm sure it's not just me! Or maybe you find it harder to learn a new skill at work, even if it's a job you've done for years? Sound familiar? That's brain fog. Some experts have described menopause brain fog as a learning problem instead of a brain problem. The SWAN trial assessed the cognitive performance of more than 2,300 people before, during, and after menopause. Researchers found that for the majority of participants, cognitive performance dipped in perimenopause and recovered in postmenopause.[45] Dr. Lisa Mosconi's research on what happens to a woman's brain as she traverses the menopause transition has shown that our brain goes through a remodeling as it adjusts and adapts to the new normal of postmenopausal hormone levels. The 30 percent dip in energy use experienced by the brain in perimenopause rebounded and even improved for many participants in postmenopause.[46] In other words, our brains learn to adjust to a new hormone soup recipe as well.

> **"My most bothersome symptom was the brain fog! I had no idea that was a symptom to expect. It has made it extremely difficult to do my job for a few months."**
> **—Laura**

The even better news is that brain fog, or subjective cognitive decline (the official medical term), does not mean you're developing dementia, even if it feels that way sometimes! Women are twice as likely as men to develop Alzheimer's disease. Indeed, some of the areas of the brain that are impacted by menopause are the same regions impacted by Alzheimer's disease. So, it's understandable that so many of us worry when we can't remember a name we've known for years and forget to pick up the one thing we needed at the grocery store. Thankfully, we know that most women will bounce back from brain fog, and researchers are studying ways to identify and reduce the risks for the small percentage of those who do develop dementia.

My mom always told me that my memory would give an elephant a run for its money, and my husband and sister often comment on my uncanny ability to remember obscure dates. So, I was understandably concerned when I suddenly started having trouble remembering why I walked into a room or which kid I needed to pick up after school. It was around my fortieth birthday that I truly felt like I was losing my mind, relying on reminders, alarms, and sticky notes to get me through my days. Here are a few notes to keep in mind:

- The fog can range from having trouble with short-term memory (names, dates, and so on) to feeling like you can't multitask as well as you used to. *Brain fog* isn't a medical term, but it's an accurate description of the changes in the ability to think clearly, concentrate, remember, or make use of new information (i.e., learn) that 60 percent of people experience during the menopause transition.[47]

- Hormone therapy may or may not help. Research suggests that some women experience short-term benefits in memory and cognition, but results of long-term studies like the Early versus Late Intervention Trial with Estradiol (ELITE), which evaluated the cognitive impact of hormone therapy after two and a half years and five years, found no impact on cognition, either negative or positive. Currently, hormone therapy is not recommended to prevent or treat cognitive decline.

- Not sleeping makes everything worse, which is why treatments that improve sleep or reduce sleep-disrupting night sweats may indirectly improve brain fog symptoms.

The Kitchen Connection

Did you know that 60 percent of your brain is made up of fat and that your brain is the hungriest organ in your body? With age and hormonal shifts, our brain's speed and efficiency can take a hit, but food and nutrition can act as system boosters, helping maintain focus, function, and clarity in menopause.

Carbohydrates Are Brain Food

Repeat after me: Glucose (from carbohydrates) is our brain and body's preferred fuel. Although the brain makes up only 2 percent of our body's weight, it uses about 20 percent of the body's total glucose-derived energy. Unlike other organs, however, the brain can't store glucose for later, so it depends on us to provide a steady supply of carbohydrates. By choosing foods rich in complex carbohydrates and fiber, we give the brain (and body) longer-lasting fuel, which is consistently linked to better overall health—including cognitive health.

Hunger fog is the difficulty we experience in decision-making when we're hungry. In one clever experiment, participants were asked questions about food, money, and other rewards under two conditions: after a meal and when they had skipped a meal. The researchers found that hunger significantly shifted people's decision-making to favor small rewards that arrived quickly rather than a larger one promised at a later time.[48] In other words, your brain can't think straight when it's hungry. I don't usually recommend eating by the clock, but it is a good idea to make sure you schedule opportunities to eat at least every few hours.

Food for Thought: Is Breakfast the Most Important Meal of the Day?

"Don't skip breakfast, it's the most important meal of the day" is something most of us have heard before. It's the reason why many schools offer a breakfast program—to ensure that all children have the chance to feed their brains before going into a classroom. For adults, skipping breakfast can increase the risk of type 2 diabetes, high blood pressure, and heart disease. Memory, problem-solving, planning, judgment, information retention, and reasoning also take a hit. And some research suggests that eating breakfast is a circadian-rhythm cue, and missing it may impact our sleep (which, in turn, may amp up the brain fog).

Building a Balanced Plate for Your Brain

The Mediterranean pattern of eating—a varied and nutrient-rich diet—probably has a role to play in the health of our brain, too. Although larger and longer trials are needed, research has found an association between the Mediterranean diet and a lower risk of mild cognitive impairment and Alzheimer's disease.[49] The MIND diet—an intervention designed to protect against neurodegenerative delay—incorporates dietary patterns from the Mediterranean and DASH diets and has been shown to promote brain health and reduce the risk of cognitive decline and neurodegenerative diseases such as Alzheimer's. The MIND diet emphasizes the following food groups:

- Leafy greens and vegetables: Greens and vegetables are rich in vitamins and minerals that support vascular health and may offer protection from oxidative stress.
- Berries: High in flavonoids, berries have anti-inflammatory and antioxidant properties.
- Nuts and olive oil: Nuts and oils contain fatty acids and polyphenols, which are anti-inflammatory and support cognitive function. In a recent study of almost a hundred thousand adults followed over twenty-eight years, eating ½ tablespoon of olive oil was associated with a 28 percent lower risk of dementia-related death compared with those who never or rarely consumed olive oil.[50]
- Whole grains and beans: Providing complex carbohydrates and fiber, beans and grains are beneficial for overall health.
- Fatty fish: These fish are a good source of omega-3 fatty acids, which are crucial for brain function and reducing inflammation.
- Lower-fat dairy: In addition to providing protein and fat, dairy provides essential nutrients like vitamin B_{12} and calcium.

You'll find many of these foods in the recipes.

A little reminder about the ketogenic (keto) diet, an ultra low-carbohydrate and high-fat diet: Although it's true that our brain can use ketones as an alternative fuel, especially during periods of reduced glucose availability (such as fasting or a keto diet), it's important to remember that ketones are the body's "break in case of emergency" fuel, not its preferred fuel source. Research is ongoing as to whether ketogenic diets may benefit conditions other than epilepsy, for which it was originally designed, but there's no evidence that ketogenic diets are superior, or even helpful otherwise.

On the Menu: Balance for Brain Health

Our brain works best when we put balance on the menu, so in addition to the obvious key ingredients +Omega-3 and +Soy & Phytoestrogens, choose foods and meals high in +Fiber to help deliver slow and steady energy to our hungry brain.

Breakfast: Tiramisu Overnight Oats (page 119)

Lunch: Ginger Squash and Red Lentil Soup (page 143)

Dinner: Sweet Potato Salmon Cakes (page 179)

Snack: Creamy Rice Pudding with Ginger and Vanilla (page 226)

Other Things to Consider

Our brain is complex and as such needs more than a to-do list to keep it healthy and working well. Although we can't always control what happens, here are a few things that may help:

MOVEMENT AND SLEEP

- Include joyful movement as often as you can, as research supports that all types of exercise are good for our brain health. Exercise gets the blood moving and helps circulate blood to the brain, and researchers are studying how strength training can improve and protect our brains as we age.
- Make sleep and managing stress a priority, as both of these can have direct and indirect effects on brain fog and brain health.

SUPPLEMENTS

- B vitamins, especially B_{12}, B_6, and folate, are in high demand by our brain, which is why some people find benefit by supplementing with a B complex vitamin.

- If eating fish several times a week isn't your thing, consider taking an omega-3 fish oil supplement that provides 1,500 mg of the omega-3 fats EPA and DHA.
- Creatine monophosphate is a compound used by muscles and the brain to make energy. This inexpensive supplement shows promise in reducing brain fog and brain health in general.

Body Changes

Body dissatisfaction and fear of weight gain are on the minds of many women before, during, and after menopause. Studies of midlife women have found that more than 60 percent of us are dissatisfied with our bodies,[51] and as few as 12 percent of women admit to being happy with what they see in the mirror.[52] In other words, you're not alone if you are bothered, baffled, and even scared by the body changes you've noticed in midlife.

> "The weight gain bothered me the most. I was surprised by feeling so lost and confused. I had zero confidence in what to eat or how to dress."
> —Trish

Let's be frank: No one looks forward to the weight gain that happens (seemingly for no reason) once we turn forty. Although I want to do this topic justice and discuss the various reasons why an overwhelming majority of people report this as one of their most bothersome symptoms in midlife, it's safe to say that weight regulation is *very* complex. It is far more than just "calories in, calories out" or eating less and moving more. Genetics, medical conditions, medications, sleep, stress, and many of the social determinants of health can play significant roles in how our bodies regulate weight.

Both men and women, across all cultures, experience changes in body shape and size due to age. However, hormonal shifts during perimenopause and menopause can accelerate these changes. Here are some things to keep in mind:

- Estimates of weight gain vary greatly, and research is quite limited. Although some data reports that the average weight change in perimenopause is in the five- to ten-pound (2.5 to 5 kg) range, I don't think we're getting the whole picture, and this may be an underestimate.

- Loss of lean muscle mass and difficulty in muscle building and maintenance are also common and can lead to changes in activity levels and energy balance.
- As we transition through to menopause, we go through a redistribution of assets, otherwise known as becoming more of an apple shape than a pear. As a result, your waistline (and maybe your bra size) may increase even if the scale doesn't change all that much.

Studies looking at menopause hormone therapy have not found that it reverses these changes, although some research does suggest that when started in perimenopause, hormone therapy may slow them down.

Weight Gain and Dieting History

Even though weight gain and body changes top the list of concerns from women in midlife, I rarely see any mention of one of the most overlooked risk factors: dieting history. Yes, you read that correctly. When I was first learning about intuitive eating, I was surprised to learn that one of the strongest predictors of future weight gain was a personal history of dieting.[53] Dieting predicts the exact thing most people start a diet to avoid. Although we don't know for certain whether it's a true cause-and-effect relationship, we do know that dieting triggers metabolic and behavioral changes to help the body regain the weight. These can include becoming more interested in eating and a drop in the fullness hormone leptin.

If you have never dieted or tried to lose a few pounds before an event or holiday, you can skip this section. But if you are like the majority of people I talk to, you have probably been on at least several different diets, if not dozens. One survey of women in the United Kingdom reported that by the age of forty-five, women had been on an average of sixty-one diets.[54] In the United States, data suggests that almost 60 percent of women report being on a diet at any given time.[55] Isn't that shocking? As Naomi Wolf states in *The Beauty Myth,* "a culture fixated on female thinness is not an obsession about female beauty, but an obsession about female obedience. Dieting is the most potent political sedative in women's history; a quietly mad population is a tractable one."[56] In my opinion, ditching diet culture is in perfect alignment with the idea of a feminist menopause.

Despite decades of research, we still don't have a long-term effective way for people to lose weight and keep it off with diet and exercise. Although most diets work in the short term, most people who lose weight will not maintain it after one year, and dieters regain on average more than half of what they lose within two years. This is true for all diets including low-carb, low-fat, or any of the other fads that promise quick and easy results. When weight is regained, it is usually regained as fat, a phenomenon sometimes referred to as fat overshooting. Because our bodies don't know the difference between intentional caloric restriction and a lack of access to food, this overshooting is thought to be protective against future periods of undernutrition.

Another unintentional side effect of weight loss is muscle loss, which is thought to be responsible for metabolic changes associated with aging and some body composition changes in menopause. When you consider a history of dieting and weight cycling with age, menopause, and age-related lean muscle changes, it is easy to see why weight changes are nearly universal among those over the age of forty.

Despite the common belief that weight gain is always bad for our health, several studies challenge this conclusion, especially for women in midlife. Midlife weight gain may offer some protection as we age by producing estrone, a type of estrogen that our tissues can use. A twenty-five-year study in Finland found that weight gain was protective against bone loss.[57] Even studies of the much-criticized body mass index (BMI) find that those with a BMI between 25 to 30 have the lowest mortality rates, further challenging the belief that a "healthy" weight can be universally defined.[58]

Even if you feel like you should lose weight, first ask yourself this question: What do you hope to achieve by losing weight? Then ask if weight loss is the only way to do that. For example, if improving health is your goal, is weight loss the only (or best) solution? The Health at Every Size (HAES) philosophy reminds us that how we live and the behaviors we choose can improve our health and reduce the risk of disease independently of what happens on the scale. And there's research to back this up. When researchers compared the health and habits of more than eleven thousand people, they found that four key behaviors—not smoking, alcohol in moderation, regular exercise, and eating five servings of fruits and vegetables per day—reduced the risk of dying regardless of BMI.[59]

Nothing is without risk in life. Although there may be risks associated with body size, we can't ignore the risks of pursuing intentional weight loss and weight cycling, either. This means that telling people to lose weight and prescribing diets to pursue this probably doesn't strike an acceptable risk-benefit ratio and shouldn't be presented as the de facto option to women in midlife.

So, instead of putting all of your time, effort, energy, and even money into trying to lose weight at any cost, why not try shifting your focus to behaviors that will support your health, regardless of what happens on the scale? This is the heart of a weight-neutral approach to health and one that I teach you how to do in this book, especially when it comes to food.

How to Support a Healthy Body Image

The number one reason that women give for wanting to lose weight is that they simply want to feel good in their skin again. I can't tell you how many women have said, "I just hate how uncomfortable I feel every day, especially when I need to get dressed or see my reflection in a mirror or photograph." Does weight loss actually improve our body image? Probably not, as people of all shapes and sizes can experience intense negative feelings about their bodies. So, if weight loss won't protect us from a negative body image, what can we do to end the body shame so many of us experience?

Intuitive Eating Is Good for Your Body Image Too

Studies show that intuitive eating reduces the likelihood of disordered eating and eating disorders and is correlated with better body image in young adults. And researchers are finding the same is likely true for older people as well. A study of two hundred women between the ages of sixty and seventy-five found that higher intuitive eating scores (determined using a validated intuitive eating scale) were associated with less restrictive eating, fewer concerns about food and body image, and fewer symptoms of depression.[60]

Know That Perimenopause May Be a Window of Vulnerability

Although body image research has mainly focused on teenagers and young women, another period of vulnerability has come to light: perimenopause. Hormonal fluctuations during this time—especially changes in estrogen and progesterone—seem to impact how women feel about their bodies. Estrogen affects many areas of the brain, so it's likely that changing hormone levels contribute to shifts in body image. Studies show that women with higher body dissatisfaction are more prone to depression, exercise less, and report a lower quality of life.[61]

How to Feel More Peaceful in Your Body Today

Even if you're not entirely convinced that weight loss won't help you with body confidence, you can use the concepts of body neutrality, body acceptance, and body appreciation to improve how you feel in your body today. Body image is how we perceive our bodies. A positive body image means seeing your body (and yourself) in a good light. A negative body image means you feel badly about your body, which can spill over into your overall self-esteem.

Body neutrality is different. It's about accepting that you are more than just your body. You don't have to love or even like your body to accept yourself. When we practice body neutrality, many of us find it easier to care for ourselves, including making healthier choices with food and exercise. If you've always tried to "hate yourself into a body you love," it's time to practice self-compassion. One great way to start is through body appreciation. Body appreciation can shift your mindset toward self-acceptance and self-compassion. Practices like gratitude journaling and body-positive affirmations help you focus on what your body does for you, rather than how it looks. A Post-it note on your bathroom mirror with the reminder "I am more than my appearance" can shift your perspective and boost both your self-esteem and your body image.

The Kitchen Connection

There's no magic recipe or plan that will change what your body looks like. As I've explained, weight regulation is complicated, and menopause adds another layer of complexity to it. My best advice for feeling good *in* and *about* your body is this:

- Nourish your body regularly with balanced plates using the gentle nutrition guidelines you're learning in this book.
- Avoid fad diets and quick fixes as they run the risk of keeping you stuck in the yo-yo cycle of weight loss and weight gain.
- Make muscle and strength your midlife priority. Include protein, joyful movement, and strength training regularly to help build and maintain muscle as you age. This is the best insurance you'll find to help keep you active and independent in midlife and beyond.

On the Menu: Body Confidence

There's more to building body confidence than just what we put on our plates. Explore ways to welcome all foods, including those containing all of the five key ingredients, and experience the confidence that comes from practicing body kindness and body respect. As you'll learn in part 3, learning to lead with satisfaction is a wonderful way to honor all types of hunger.

Breakfast: Savory Sweet Potato Egg Bites (page 129)

Lunch: Savory Sweet Potato, Chickpea, and Peanut Stew (page 151)

Dinner: Spinach and Mozzarella Pita Pizza (page 155)

Snack: No-Bake Peanut Butter Chocolate Tofu Pie (page 229)

Genitourinary Health

During menopause, the drop in estrogen impacts our pelvic floor, urethra, bladder, vulva, and vagina. It's not just about lubrication, either, as changes in tissue elasticity and vaginal flora explain why up to 70 percent of us will experience symptoms such as burning and itching, vaginal dryness, painful sex, and urinary symptoms including burning, frequency, and urgency in postmenopause.[62] Collectively, these symptoms are recognized as the genitourinary syndrome of menopause (GSM)—and it's no joke. This collection of symptoms is the result of the decline in estrogen and other hormones during menopause. And, contrary to what you may think, sex is the least important reason to treat it. The impact of GSM on quality of life goes beyond the bathroom and bedroom, contributing to decreased self-esteem and

"I spent months trying to treat what I thought was a stubborn bladder infection. I wish I'd known that my symptoms were caused by low estrogen, even though I wasn't experiencing vaginal dryness." —Amelia

relationship stress.[63] Many women experience reduced quality of life and even increased rates of depression and anxiety. And many of the women I speak to feel embarrassed or reluctant to discuss these symptoms with their health-care providers—all the more reason to shed more light on what you might experience.

- As estrogen levels decline, vaginal dryness and discomfort become more common and many experience painful intercourse and discomfort with regular activities like walking or riding a bike.
- Changes in the vaginal tissue can also lead to more infections of the vulva, vagina, urethra, and bladder.
- Urinary frequency, urgency, dribbling, and incontinence are more common.
- Vaginal moisturizers can be helpful, but many people respond better when topical estrogen is used as well. Others may require systemic hormone therapy.
- The use of water- or silicone-based lubricants is recommended to increase pleasure and reduce discomfort with intercourse.

There's some evidence that soy foods and phytoestrogens can help with vaginal dryness and discomfort, but none that compares to the effectiveness of topical estrogen. The standard treatments for the symptoms of GSM include local estrogen therapy, as either a cream, tablet, or ring. This helps to replenish estrogen in the affected tissues, alleviating symptoms. Research assures us that local estrogen is safe for almost everyone, including those with a history of breast cancer (though you'll want to discuss it with your doctor, of course). A few countries have made the progressive move to make vaginal estrogen therapy available over the counter, but many countries, including the United States and Canada, require a prescription.

The Kitchen Connection

You'd be forgiven for not thinking about the health of your genitourinary tract while planning your meals. But food and nutrition do have roles to play here, even if they're not as obvious as with hot flashes or mood swings.

On the Menu: Vaginal Health

Nutrition isn't leading the charge with genitourinary health, but it still has an important role to play. Choose foods and meals that will help keep you hydrated, and it won't hurt to add foods from the key ingredient +Soy & Phytoestrogens.

Breakfast: Blueberry Banana Tofu Smoothie (page 234)

Lunch: Thai Lentil and Sweet Potato Soup (page 139)

Dinner: Marinated Tofu and Soba Noodles with Bok Choy (page 183)

Snack: Citrus and Honey Summer Spritzer (page 239)

Stay Hydrated

Although it might seem obvious, staying hydrated can help maintain vaginal health during menopause. As estrogen levels decline, the vaginal tissues become thinner and less elastic and produce less natural lubrication. Proper hydration helps support overall vaginal health in several ways:

- **Tissue hydration:** Adequate water intake helps keep vaginal tissues moist and supple, reducing the risk of irritation and discomfort.
- **Mucus production:** Hydration supports the body's ability to produce mucus, which is essential for maintaining vaginal lubrication.
- **Balanced pH:** Staying hydrated helps maintain the vagina's natural acidic environment, which is crucial for preventing infections and maintaining a healthy microbiome.
- **Skin elasticity:** Well-hydrated skin, including the vulvar area, maintains better elasticity and is less prone to irritation and microtears.

How much water do you need? Experts no longer recommend hard-and-fast rules but instead recommend letting your thirst levels guide you. That being said, you may find it helpful to keep a water bottle nearby to help you remember to drink.

Keep Your Microbiome Well Fed

Many people have heard of the gut microbiome, the population of microorganisms that live in our digestive tract. We also have a vaginal microbiome, which is dominated by the bacterial species *Lactobacillus*. Anyone who has experienced a vaginal yeast infection (i.e., thrush) knows what happens when this balance gets thrown off. During menopause, hormonal shifts can lead to changes in the vaginal tissues. Estrogen helps maintain the thickness and elasticity of the vaginal lining, and it supports an environment that encourages *Lactobacillus* to thrive. When estrogen levels fall, the vaginal tissues may thin, become drier, and lose some of their acidity, making it easier for harmful bacteria and yeast to take over.

This is where fermented foods come in. Consuming probiotic-rich foods like yogurt, kefir, sauerkraut, and miso can help support the microbial balance in the body, potentially benefiting the vaginal microbiome as well. Although more research is needed specifically on fermented foods and the vaginal microbiome, many women find that supporting gut health with probiotic foods helps support their genitourinary health in menopause.

Moisturize, Moisturize, Moisturize

If you experience external dryness and itching around the vulva, you probably have an effective topical moisturizer sitting in your kitchen cupboard. Coconut oil and olive oil are inexpensive, unscented, and readily available. But, if your nose scrunches up just thinking about sharing a product between your bathroom and kitchen, I'd suggest buying separate bottles. I've been recommending coconut oil as a moisturizer for years, in part because it's solid at room temperature and easy to apply. Other nonhormonal options include topical hyaluronic acid, over-the-counter vaginal moisturizers, and lubricants. These can provide symptomatic relief, but keep in mind that moisturizers do not treat the physical changes to the tissues seen with menopause; they simply keep the skin moisturized.

Heart Health

If menopause were a Broadway show, hot flashes and mood swings would be the lead roles, stealing the spotlight. However, just like in any stage production, much is happening backstage and behind the curtain. We must keep the big picture in mind to understand how midlife hormonal changes impact our overall health, especially in the long term. Cardiovascular disease (CVD) is an umbrella term for conditions affecting the heart and blood vessels. The most common is coronary heart disease (CHD), commonly referred to as heart disease, describing the blockage of arteries that can result in a heart attack or stroke. Atherosclerosis, the development of plaque in the arteries leading to blockage, is something we can impact with nutrition and lifestyle.

> "My doctor and I were so focused on my hot flashes and insomnia that we didn't notice the jump in my cholesterol and blood pressure. I was surprised how much had changed in just a couple of years."
> —Erin

You might be surprised to learn that heart disease, not breast cancer, is the leading cause of death in women, affecting one out of every three women.[64] Although it's viewed as a disease primarily affecting men, the rates of heart disease equalize between the sexes by our mid-fifties. It's important to note that the timing of menopause affects this, as the loss of estrogen is a contributing factor; estrogen helps keep cholesterol, blood sugar, and blood pressure in healthy ranges. This isn't all bad news, though, since heart disease takes many years to develop. Knowing a window of opportunity exists can empower you to manage your risk factors.

How Menopause and Estrogen Impact Heart Health

Midlife brings a convergence of risk factors, including age-related increases in blood sugar and blood pressure, and lesser-known risk factors like premature menopause and pregnancy history. A large study of more than five hundred thousand women in the United Kingdom found that early menarche (before age ten), early menopause (before forty-five), earlier age at first birth, and having a history of miscarriage, stillbirth, or hysterectomy also increased the risk of heart disease.[65]

Cholesterol and Triglycerides

When estrogen levels decline sharply around late perimenopause, cholesterol levels often jump. This increase applies to total cholesterol levels as well as the presence of low-density lipoprotein (LDL), the so-called bad cholesterol. In fact, an increase of 10 to 15 percent in cholesterol levels, especially in the year following the last menstrual period, is common. Although these are potentially frightening statistics, knowing that these changes are coming down the pike can provide comfort. For instance, you can use this opportunity to increase your intake of fiber and plant-based protein, two gentle nutrition approaches.

Triglyceride levels may also rise in menopause. Although triglycerides are a major source of energy for the body, high levels are considered a risk factor for diabetes and heart and liver disease. When we consume more energy than our body needs in the moment (regardless of its source), the excess energy is converted into triglycerides and stored in fat cells. Later, hormones regulate the release of triglycerides for energy between meals. There are also genetic causes of high triglycerides, so knowing your family history is important.

WHAT'S NORMAL?
UNDERSTANDING YOUR CHOLESTEROL LEVELS

Lipid Profile Component	US Reference Values (mg/dL)	Canadian Reference Values (mmol/L)
Total cholesterol	Less than 200	Less than 5.2
LDL (Low-density lipoprotein)	Less than 100	Less than 2.6
HDL (High-density lipoprotein)	60 or higher	1.55 or higher
Triglycerides	Less than 150	Less than 1.7

Your doctor may do additional testing to help assess your individual heart disease risk. Lipoprotein (a) (Lp[a]) is a type of lipoprotein that has been identified as an independent risk factor for cardiovascular diseases, and elevated levels of Lp(a) are associated with atherosclerosis. Apolipoprotein B (apoB) is another type of protein found in LDL cholesterol and is linked to the transport of cholesterol into artery walls and the development of plaque that leads to atherosclerosis. While neither of these are usually included in regular screenings for cholesterol, it's worth discussing them with your doctor, especially if you have a family history of heart disease.

Blood Pressure

High blood pressure, or hypertension, becomes more common in midlife and menopause. It's a good idea to regularly check your blood pressure, as most people won't have symptoms. Normal blood pressure is 120/80, and it's considered high at 140/90. If your blood pressure is between these ranges, it's an opportunity to make changes to bring it back into the healthy range.

Blood Sugar, Insulin Resistance, and Diabetes

Insulin resistance and its impact on heart health during menopause are hot topics. You may have read or heard these attention-grabbing opinions:

> "Midlife weight gain is caused by insulin resistance."
>
> "Hormonal imbalance is the cause of meno-belly."
>
> "All women in menopause have insulin resistance."
>
> "Women over forty need to avoid carbs because of insulin resistance."

Here's what we do know: Menopause *is* associated with an increased risk of both insulin resistance and type 2 diabetes. What we don't know is whether menopause (and the loss of estrogen) is the sole underlying cause. Yes, estrogen does indeed influence insulin sensitivity, but we know it's not the only factor because although every woman will go through menopause, not everyone will develop insulin resistance or diabetes. A large Chinese study also uncovered a link between age at menopause and diabetes, finding that the risk was highest in women who experienced menopause before the age of forty, and lowest for those who went through menopause between the ages of forty-five and forty-nine.[66] This association was recently confirmed in a large study that compared the data from thirteen studies, reiterating the importance of identifying those at risk for early and premature menopause.[67] Other changes during menopause, including aging and decreased muscle mass, likely contribute to insulin resistance and diabetes risk as well.

Much research has been published on the relationships among sugar, carbohydrates, and diabetes. You can be assured that eating carbohydrates doesn't cause diabetes. In fact, research has found that eating carbohydrates, even in the range of 45 to 65 percent of total caloric intake is not associated with an increased risk of developing type 2 diabetes.[68] This topic is often misunderstood, so I'm going to use a car's engine as an analogy to explain it.

A car's engine burns gas and produces energy to power the car. Similarly, our bodies use food as fuel for our cells to produce energy. Insulin acts like a valve that allows fuel to enter the engine. When everything works well, the fuel (glucose) is burned efficiently in the engine (cells), powering the car (body). When we run into engine trouble (insulin resistance), the valves (insulin) get sticky and stop the smooth flow of fuel into the engine. The engine (cells) becomes less efficient, producing less energy. Eventually, if the problem worsens, the engine may stop being able to accept fuel altogether, which is like the body developing diabetes, where it can't manage glucose without external help.

If Your Blood Sugar Needs a Tune-Up

If you're managing rising blood sugars or have been told you have prediabetes or insulin resistance, here are some gentle nutrition suggestions:

- Make regular and paced deliveries of fuel: Arrange time for regular meals that allow you to eat when you experience comfortable hunger, a sign that your engine wants fuel. A study of people with type 2 diabetes in Brazil found that, regardless of body size, people with higher intuitive eating scores were significantly more likely to have better glycemic control.[69]
- Build balanced plates that include carbohydrates, protein, and fat, a combination that delivers slow and steady fuel.
- Emphasize adding the key ingredients +Fiber and +Protein to your plate as they will help slow the rise in blood sugar after a meal.
- Do some engine maintenance: Muscle cells are your engine's number one customer, requiring a lot of fuel on a regular basis. Using your muscles, even just by walking for fifteen minutes after a meal, can improve your blood sugar.[70] Using more muscles requires more energy, which results in the engine getting a tune-up to meet the demand. In other words, try something new and welcome joyful movement in new-to-you and fun ways.

Diet and wellness culture would lead you to believe that the fuel source (usually carbs) is the problem and that using another fuel source (usually fat or protein) will fix the problem. Although you might experience short-term improvements in blood sugar by switching fuels, it doesn't address the real root of the problem: the engine. Insulin resistance doesn't mean you aren't making enough insulin; it means that the cells in your muscles, fat, and liver aren't responding to insulin, thereby prompting your pancreas to make more insulin to compensate. As a result, both insulin and blood sugar levels are elevated. To use our car analogy, insulin resistance is the check engine light, and you should probably pull over and see your mechanic.

There is no single food that causes or cures diabetes. There are patterns of eating (e.g., high fiber) that positively influence blood sugar and diabetes, but using words like *good* and *bad* to describe foods isn't helpful and makes it harder to stay out of the diet mentality. One last thing to remember: Insulin resistance is a symptom, not a disease. And it is not a moral failing caused by your body size or shape—or a sign that you don't care about your health.

On the Menu: Heart Health

Using a plant-forward approach makes it easy to choose foods that are both delicious and good for our hearts. A menu designed with lowering cholesterol in mind would be well served by including recipes from the +Soy & Phytoestrogens and +Fiber sections. Both of these are also helpful if you have high blood sugar or diabetes, along with +Protein recipes.

Breakfast: Pumpkin Smoothie Bowl (page 126)

Lunch: Beet and Pomegranate Couscous (page 203)

Dinner: Pasta with Rustic Red Lentil Marinara Sauce (page 158)

Snack: Banana Flax Muffins (page 218)

Food for Thought: How Heart Healthy Is a Glass of Wine?

For years, people have been told that a glass of red wine with dinner is considered good for the heart. This idea was eagerly adopted in the 1990s as one of the secrets of longevity enjoyed by the French. However, new research has highlighted that the risks of regularly drinking alcohol outweigh the benefits. Although it's true that red wine is rich in polyphenols and antioxidants, drinking alcohol can also increase blood pressure, triglycerides, and the risk of many cancers. I recommend following the low-risk drinking guidelines for women to consume fewer than seven standard drinks per week. Some countries, like Canada, have updated their guidelines and now define low-risk as staying under two drinks per week.

The Kitchen Connection

Heart health is a long game, with eating patterns mattering more than individual foods. Not surprisingly, diets that lower heart disease risk are lower in saturated fats, higher in fiber, and include plant-based protein, whole grains, fruits, and vegetables. The Mediterranean diet's nonrestrictive and plant-forward approach meets these criteria.

Plants

I love beans and lentils because they make it easy and delicious to add more protein and fiber to your meals. Soy is a notable player in this game, too—and not just because of its isoflavones. Eating 25 g of soy protein per day can lower cholesterol levels by as much as 4 to 6 percent.[71] And unfermented soy products, including tofu, soy milk, edamame, and soy nuts and sprouts, can reduce total cholesterol and triglycerides and improve levels of HDL cholesterol.[72]

Dietary Fat

Fat is one of the essential macronutrients our bodies use for energy. It helps increase the absorption of fat-soluble nutrients and makes food more delicious and satisfying. Saturated fats come almost exclusively from animal foods and are most associated with high cholesterol and heart disease. Unsaturated fats are classified as either monounsaturated or polyunsaturated. Monounsaturated fats are found in foods such as olives, avocados, and peanuts while polyunsaturated fats (which include essential omega-3s and omega-6s) come from foods like flax, fish, and walnuts. Walnuts, flax, and hemp seeds supply alpha-linolenic acid (ALA), a precursor to omega-3s that our body can use to reduce inflammation and the risk of heart disease. Although unsaturated fats offer several health benefits, it's important to lead with satisfaction when making dietary changes to avoid all-or-nothing thinking. You don't need to eliminate foods rich in saturated fat; instead, focus on adding foods with unsaturated fats more often.

Dietary Cholesterol

I've got good news for you if you've shied away from eggs because of cholesterol concerns. Although dietary cholesterol was once thought to play a major role in cholesterol levels and heart disease, research now shows that the cholesterol our body produces naturally in our liver has a much greater impact on blood cholesterol levels. This means that for most people, eating foods with cholesterol, like eggs, won't cause your cholesterol levels to jump. Also, cholesterol, like saturated fat, is found only in foods that come from animals. So, if you're eating a diet lower in saturated fats, you'll likely be reducing your intake of dietary cholesterol, too.

Fiber

Fiber is the secret sauce to supporting heart health—it not only helps lower cholesterol but also supports healthy blood sugar levels. For example, getting 10 g of soluble fiber (i.e., viscous fiber) per day can reduce cholesterol levels by up to 10 percent.[73] We'll cover fiber in detail on page 95, when we get to the section on the key ingredients.

Sodium and Potassium

Sodium and potassium are essential minerals that play important roles in maintaining heart health, especially during menopause when blood pressure naturally tends to rise due to increasing salt sensitivity. High intake of sodium can cause water retention, which increases blood volume and, subsequently, blood pressure, so it's a good idea to choose reduced-salt options when you can. Does the type of salt make a difference? Is pink salt from the Himalayas really better for us? Probably not. Although these salts do come with higher levels of trace minerals, the sodium content is the same. Potassium, on the other hand, helps counteract the effects of sodium. It aids in relaxing blood vessel walls and helps the body excrete sodium, thereby lowering blood pressure. Potassium is found in a wide variety of foods, including bananas, oranges, spinach, sweet potatoes, and avocados.

Bone Health

A woman's risk of breaking a hip is equal to her combined risk of breast, uterine, and ovarian cancer. One in five women who break a hip will not survive the first year.[74] Do I have your attention now? Good! Even though we reach peak bone mass in our early thirties, long before menopause, you can start learning how to take care of your bones.

In our thirties and forties, we gradually start to lose bone density at a rate of 1 to 2 percent a year. This loss speeds up as we approach menopause, with an estimated 10 to 20 percent of bone density lost during the menopause transition, significantly increasing the risk of osteoporosis.[75] People who experience premature ovarian insufficiency or early menopause may be at even higher risk. Osteoporosis is when bone mineral density and bone mass decrease, leading to a loss of bone strength that can increase the risk of fractures. One in ten women over the age of sixty are affected, and it's shocking to realize that worldwide, one in three women over the age of fifty will experience a fracture due to osteoporosis.

> **"My grandmother broke her hip at her seventy-fifth birthday party. Even though she lived for several more years, my family has always said that Grandma's life ended at seventy-five because she was never the same after that. I want to avoid that at all costs."**
> **—Fiona**

If you've had a bone density scan (DEXA scan) to check the strength of your bones, you may have been told you have osteopenia. This means some loss of bone density but not enough to be classified as osteoporosis. Many women are surprised and worried when diagnosed with osteopenia, concerned about their future health and independence. The good news is that it's never too late to make an impact on bone density and reduce your risk of a fall or fracture.

Osteoporosis is often a silent disease, discovered only after a bone fracture. Some risk factors for osteoporosis are modifiable while others are not. You can't change your family history, whether you were born with a uterus, or your height and frame. However, you can influence certain behaviors, such as smoking, alcohol consumption, calcium intake, and physical activity. If you're curious about your risks, these tools are available and free to access:

- **Know Your Bones:** An online tool from Healthy Bones Australia and the Garvan Institute of Medical Research that helps assess fracture risk, including for those with osteopenia and osteoporosis
- **FRAX:** A widely used fracture risk assessment tool developed by the University of Sheffield, estimating an individual's ten-year probability of fracture based on risk factors
- **Osteoporosis Risk Assessment Instrument (ORAI):** A simple scoring tool that identifies women at risk for osteoporosis by assessing age, weight, and current estrogen use

The Kitchen Connection

By menopause, the peak bone density ship has sailed, and the focus is now on maintaining as much bone density as possible, slowing the rate of bone loss, and reducing the risk of falling with strength, mobility, and balance training. Contrary to common belief, it is possible to build bone density during menopause. Bone is constantly being made and broken down. Our goal is to provide the necessary ingredients and tools for its health.

Calcium

Many women are confused about calcium. Make no mistake, calcium is crucial for bone health, with a recommended daily intake for postmenopausal women typically around 1,200 mg. Dairy products like milk, cheese, and yogurt are excellent sources. For those who are lactose intolerant or prefer nondairy options, fortified plant-based milks, leafy green vegetables, almonds, and tofu are great alternatives.

Vitamin D

Vitamin D increases calcium absorption in the intestine. Although sunlight exposure helps produce vitamin D, many people need supplements to meet the recommended intake, usually around 1,000 IU per day. Foods rich in vitamin D include fatty fish such as salmon and mackerel, egg yolks, certain mushrooms, and fortified foods like milk and orange juice. Try the Sweet Potato Salmon Cakes (page 179), which uses canned salmon rich in calcium, protein, and vitamin D. Your bones will thank you for it!

Protein

Adequate protein intake helps keep muscles strong, supporting and protecting bones. Some studies have found that protein can have a positive effect on bone density, but others have not. Some have even found that bone density is negatively affected by high levels of protein, although a recent review from the National Osteoporosis Foundation found that protein intake of 25 to 30 percent of total energy intake has no negative effects on bone health.[76]

Magnesium and Vitamin K

Magnesium and vitamin K play supporting roles in bone health. Magnesium helps convert vitamin D into its active form, which aids calcium absorption. Foods rich in magnesium include nuts, seeds, whole grains, and leafy green vegetables. Vitamin K is involved in bone metabolism and can be found in leafy greens, broccoli, and Brussels sprouts. A particular type of vitamin K, called K_2 or sometimes MK_4, gained popularity a few years ago for its possible role in bone strength. That said, studies are limited and results have been mixed. Until new research is available, supplementing is not recommended at this time, but food sources can always be included. These mainly include fermented sources, including natto (fermented soybeans), aged cheese, egg yolks, and butter.

Isoflavones

The Shanghai Women's Health Study (SWHS) was the first large study to report on the association between soy food intake and fracture risk. Researchers found that consuming soy was linked to a significantly lower risk of fractures, especially in women early in their postmenopausal years.[77] Since then, studies on soy protein and isoflavone supplements in postmenopausal women have had mixed results. Some clinical trials show that soy offers significant protection for bone density while others show little to no effect. Although I don't recommend comparing the bone-boosting effects of soy or isoflavones with the well-known benefits of hormone therapy (especially estrogen), I *do* welcome any additional benefits they impart as a bonus!

On the Menu: Strong Bones

Although choosing foods rich in +Calcium may seem obvious, paying attention to +Protein and +Soy & Phytoestrogens foods is just as important. Along with joyful movement, these foods can help your bones weather the changes that come with menopause.

Breakfast: Key Lime Overnight Oats (page 115)

Lunch: Mushroom Lentil Stew (page 147)

Dinner: Spinach and Mozzarella Pita Pizza (page 155)

Snack: Tofu Pudding (page 223)

Other Things to Consider

There's more to bone health than what's on your plate. Movement and exercise, along with hormones, can help reduce the risk of osteoporosis in menopause.

MOVEMENT

- Weight-bearing exercises like walking, jogging, and dancing, along with resistance training, are crucial for bone health. These activities stimulate bone growth, improving strength, mobility, and balance, thus reducing fall risk. Experts recommend two to three days per week of strength training along with other weight-bearing activities like walking. Work with a personal trainer if you are new to strength training, have osteoporosis, or have other health concerns.
- Activities such as tai chi, yoga, and Pilates can enhance balance, coordination, and flexibility. Simple practices like standing on one leg while brushing your teeth or doing gentle stretches can also make a difference in bone health and are just as important as picking up a dumbbell.

HORMONE THERAPY

- Hormone therapy has been shown to have a significant impact in this area, especially for those who have additional risk factors for osteoporosis such as early or premature menopause. When estrogen levels drop during menopause, bone resorption (the process where bone is broken down and its minerals released into the blood) accelerates, leading to a decrease in bone density. Prevention of osteoporosis and fractures is one of the Menopause Society's indications for using hormone therapy.

Undiet It! Ditching the Diet Is Good for Your Bones

There's a side effect of dieting that's not often mentioned but deserves our full attention: Dieting often leads to loss of lean muscle and bone density. A study of 101 postmenopausal women placed on either a moderate or severe supervised diet for one year found that both groups had significant decreases in whole-body lean mass, and 40 percent of dieters in the severe group developed osteopenia. Interestingly, the decrease in bone mineral density continued in the severe group, even after weight loss plateaued after six months. This occurred despite ensuring adequate dietary protein (1 g/kg) and despite the fact that the meal replacement products used provided more than the recommended dietary intake for vitamin D and calcium for women aged fifty-one to seventy.[78]

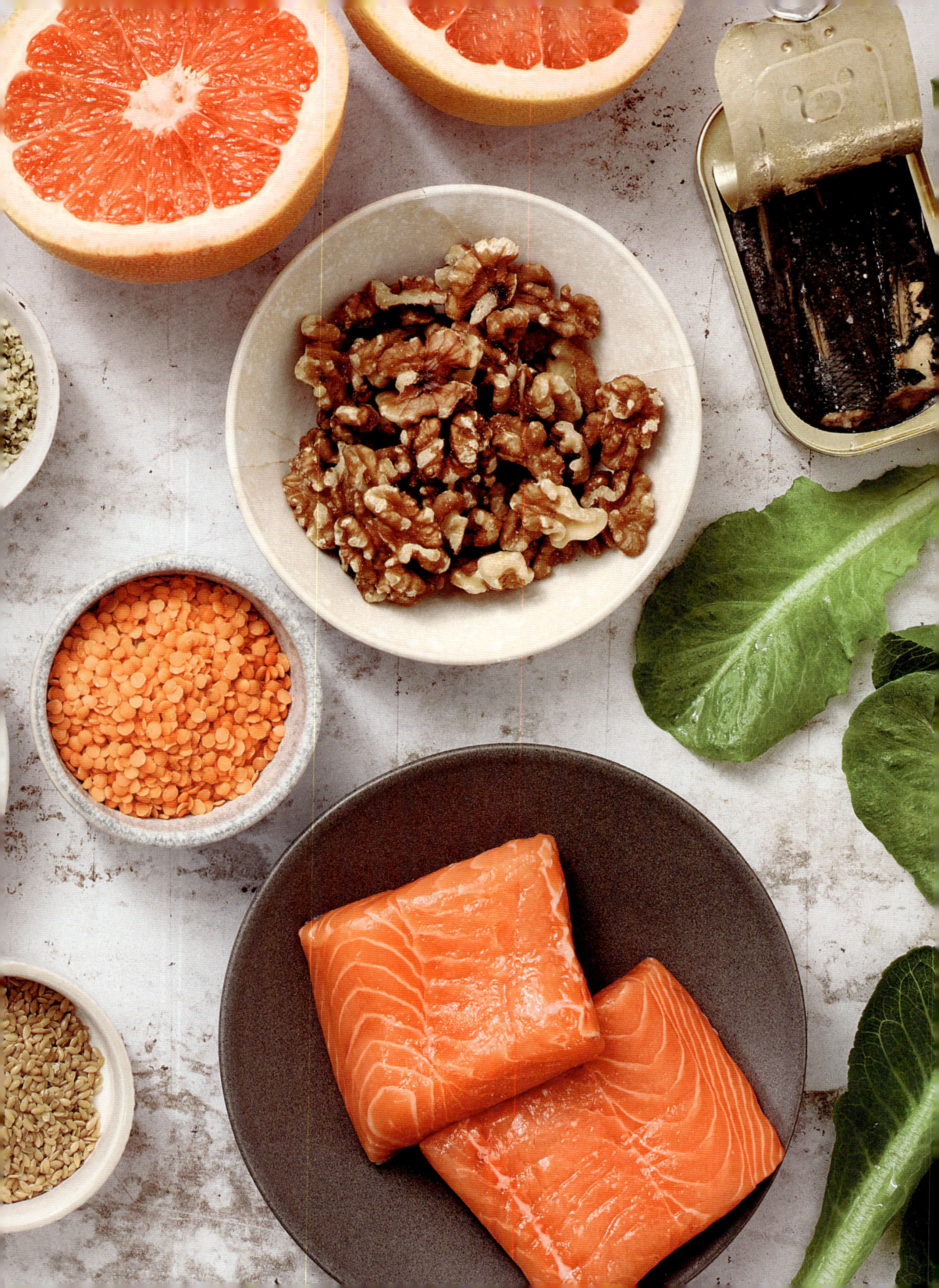

PART 3

The Foundations of a Nourished Menopause

Here is the fun part, putting into practice what you've learned about managing menopause with delicious food in easy and intuitive ways. It's time to get to know the **five key ingredients**: soy and phytoestrogens, protein, fiber, calcium, and omega-3s. These ingredients represent simplicity and versatility, not superiority. Each has a role to play in our overall health but may also be connected to a symptom, specific health concern, or both. My goal isn't to give you the impression that any of these are superfoods, but rather that many needs can be met by regularly including these ingredients. In other words, these key ingredients give you a big bang for your buck.

The Basics of Building a Nutrition Capsule Wardrobe

A standard menopause nutrition capsule wardrobe will include all of the key ingredients as each fit the pattern of eating that will help manage symptoms and provide what is needed for a healthy heart, strong bones, and sharp mind. Similarly, what yours looks like will vary depending on tastes, preferences, and needs.

Lead with Satisfaction

When it comes to nutrition, what you want is just as important as what you need! Welcome the pleasure of eating by putting satisfaction first. Do you want something hot or cold? Soft or crunchy? Sweet or savory? When you make satisfaction a priority, you avoid falling into the scarcity trap and will find it easier to listen to your fullness cues and feel satisfied. What about foods that taste good but don't necessarily have a lot of nutrient density? You can still lead with satisfaction and use the nutrition by addition philosophy to build a balanced plate, by adding foods instead of taking them away. Moderation will feel much easier when you learn to say yes instead of no.

Build a Solid Foundation

Plan to include protein, carbohydrates, and fats at most meals. These are like the timeless and iconic pieces in your closet that never go out of style and will never let you down. How much of each you'll need depends on your personal needs and preferences, and can change from day to day. Recall the image of the three-legged stool (page 13) and make sure the foundation you build can support the seat of your stool. A common myth about food is that our nutrition needs are static. The truth is that they're quite dynamic, in sync with your body's need for energy. You can honor your health with gentle nutrition by learning to listen and respond to your hunger and fullness cues and find the sweet spot between what you want and what you need.

What Is Gentle Nutrition?

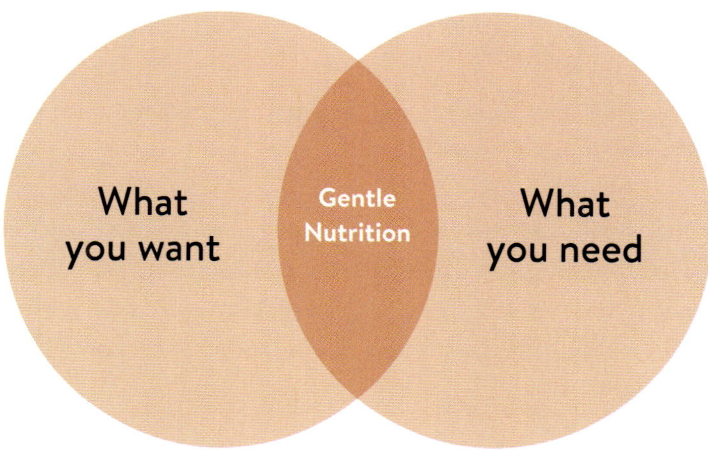

Layer in Your Key Ingredients

When building a capsule wardrobe with clothing, you look for versatile pieces that can adapt to your needs. The five key ingredients are the versatile pieces in your meal plan. And just like the reliable little black dress that you can dress up or dress down, I hope you'll find many new favorite recipes in these pages as you learn how to make menopause nutrition feel straightforward and intuitive. To make it easier, you'll find tags on the recipes highlighting which key ingredients are featured, allowing you to quickly choose recipes that meet your individual needs. For example:

- If you are experiencing many symptoms of menopause, especially hot flashes and night sweats, choose recipes with the +Soy & Phytoestrogens tag. You can look at the "Help Me Quickly Hot Flash Meal Plan!" (page 242) for ideas.

- If lowering your cholesterol and heart health are priorities, include recipes with the tags +Soy & Phytoestrogens, +Fiber, and +Omega-3.
- To support blood sugar and metabolic health, choose more recipes that feature +Fiber and +Protein.
- For a bone health focus, prioritize recipes and foods with +Calcium.
- If you're working on building muscle and strength, you'll want to include recipes with +Protein.
- If you want to prioritize satiety and satisfaction, try adding recipes with +Fiber and +Protein.

If you're wondering why I haven't included a breakdown of each recipe's nutrition, it's because I'm not convinced that knowing exact amounts of the nutrients in our food is helpful. Perhaps more importantly, I don't think we need to count, measure, or track every calorie or gram to support a nourished menopause.

Key Ingredient: Soy and Phytoestrogens

I often call soy foods and phytoestrogens a midlife gal's best friends, regardless of whether you're experiencing hot flashes or not. Although it's true that foods rich in isoflavones, the type of phytoestrogen found in soy foods, may help keep you cool, it's far from the only reason you'll want to enjoy them.

WHY SOY AND PHYTOESTROGENS ARE KEY INGREDIENTS IN MENOPAUSE

- Consuming 25 to 50 mg of soy isoflavones per day may help tame hot flash frequency and severity.
- Enjoying 25 g of soy protein per day can reduce cholesterol levels (about 4 to 8 percent) and therefore the risk of heart disease.[1]
- Soy foods and phytoestrogen-rich foods may improve cognitive function, memory, sleep, and mood.[2]
- Phytoestrogen-rich foods are safe and likely protective against many types of cancer, including breast cancer.

Types of Phytoestrogens

Phytoestrogens bear a slight resemblance to the hormone estrogen. Fortunately for us, it's this unique feature that can help support some of the symptoms we experience in perimenopause and menopause, along with reducing some of the risks to our overall health in postmenopause. If you are one of the many women for whom hormone therapy has offered a safe and effective solution to hot flashes and night sweats, great. But if hormone therapy hasn't worked, or isn't an option for you, you'll be happy to know that phytoestrogens may help. Although phytoestrogens aren't as potent as our own estrogen, their ability to selectively and weakly bind to our estrogen receptors explains why many people, including me, have found relief from hot flashes and night sweats by including foods such as soy, flax, beans, and legumes in their diets. Phytoestrogens come in several forms, but the three main types are isoflavones, coumestans, and lignans.

Isoflavones: The Soy Sensation

Nearly forty years ago, researchers noted that women in Asian countries had very different experiences in menopause compared to those in North America. In the 1980s, surveys of women living in Japan found that they experienced very few of the typical perimenopause and menopause symptoms. Hot flashes and night sweats were among the least reported symptoms, unlike in North American and European studies. At the time, many theories were proposed, including the possibility that the term *hot flash* simply didn't have an equivalent meaning in Japanese culture. However, subsequent research suggested a dietary link between soy intake in the traditional Japanese diet and fewer menopausal symptoms.

Isoflavones are primarily found in soy foods like tofu, edamame, and soy milk. The two most common types, daidzein and genistein, have a particular affinity for the estrogen receptor beta (ER-β), located in various tissues, including the brain, bones, and blood vessels. When isoflavones bind to ER-β, they produce a mild estrogen-like effect, which can help relieve symptoms like hot flashes and night sweats in some women.

Unlike the stronger estrogen receptor alpha (ER-α), the interaction with ER-β is considered protective. It provides some of estrogen's benefits without raising the risk of estrogen-related conditions, such as breast cancer. This is one reason soy and isoflavones are considered safe for most people. Chickpeas also contain isoflavones, but more research is needed to determine if chickpea isoflavones offer similar phytoestrogenic effects.

Here's an example of how to eat a minimum of 25 g of soy protein and 50 mg of isoflavones:

1 cup (240 ml) of soy milk = 8 g of soy protein and 20–25 mg of isoflavones

⅓ cup (30 g) of soy nuts = 10 g of soy protein and 45 mg of isoflavones

½ cup (80 g) of shelled edamame = 10 g of soy protein and 16 mg of isoflavones

ISOFLAVONE CONTENT OF SOY FOODS	
Soybeans (mature) (⅔ cup/100 g)	65
Tempeh (3½ ounces/100 g)	61
Soy nuts (⅓ cup/30 g)	45
Tofu (3½ ounces/100 g)	30
Edamame, cooked (1 cup/160 g)	32
Soy milk (1 cup/240 ml)	25
Soy yogurt (½ cup/120 g)	21

Lignans and Coumestans: A Gift from Whole Grains, Beans, and Seeds

Lignans are found in grains and seeds, including flax. Although they don't directly bind to estrogen receptors like isoflavones, the metabolites created during the digestive process can still influence estrogen activity. Coumestans are found in food such as split peas, pinto beans, lima beans, and especially alfalfa and clover sprouts. Coumestan-rich diets containing vegetables, fruits, and whole grains may offer protection from heart disease and some types of cancer.[3]

The Safety of Phytoestrogens

Phytoestrogens have an excellent safety profile. For most women, phytoestrogen-rich foods like soybeans, tofu, and flax are safe and beneficial to eat during and after menopause. Many women worry about soy affecting thyroid function, but recent research shows soy foods do not impact thyroid function.[4] The same is true for breast cancer. Large, long-term studies consistently show that women who regularly eat soy have a lower risk of breast cancer. Some studies suggest that soy may even reduce the risk of breast cancer recurrence.[5]

The most extensive study on soy and breast cancer risk, the Shanghai Women's Health Study, included more than seventy-three thousand women followed for seven years. The study found that women who ate the most soy had nearly a 60 percent lower risk of breast cancer. These results were confirmed in a follow-up study seven years later.[6] Similar conclusions were drawn from studies of breast cancer survivors in the United States and Canada, confirming that women who ate more soy had a lower risk of recurrence and death.[7] In other words, soy foods are very safe.

The Recipe for Adding Soy and Phytoestrogens to Your Plate

Regardless of your hot flash status, women should find ways to regularly enjoy soy and phytoestrogen-rich foods. As you learned in part 2, they are a staple ingredient for managing several menopausal symptoms and can help keep our heart healthy.

Make the Switch to Soy Milk

The easiest place to start is using soy milk in place of your usual milk. Although brands may vary, 1 cup (240 ml) of soy milk typically provides about 8 g of protein and 20 to 25 mg of isoflavones. You can use soy milk in smoothies, on cereal, or to add creaminess to soup. You'll find many recipes in this book that use soy milk, so I recommend starting with the Carrot Cake Overnight Oats (page 117) or the Chia Seed Pudding (page 225) if soy milk is new to you.

Snack on Soy

Two of my favorite soy snacks are soy nuts and edamame. You can find plain and seasoned soy nuts in most health food stores, which can be enjoyed on their own or to add crunch and satisfaction to a salad. One-third of a cup (30 g) soy nuts boasts 10 g of protein and an impressive 45 mg of isoflavones. Edamame is easy to prepare at home as well, especially since frozen edamame is widely available. Simply bring water to a boil and stir in the edamame with a pinch of salt. Cook for four to five minutes. Drain, season with salt if desired, and serve. You can also cook edamame in a microwave: Add 2 tablespoons of water per 1 cup (160 g) of edamame and heat for three to four minutes in a covered dish.

Nutrition by Addition

You can enjoy the benefits of soy and phytoestrogens without committing to an entirely meatless meal. Add a tablespoon of flax to yogurt or a handful of shelled edamame to a stir-fry with chicken or meat. Saucy Slow-Cooked Tikka Masala (page 163) is a tasty example of how chicken and chickpeas are a great combination.

Key Ingredient: Protein

In addition to building and maintaining muscle, protein also helps stabilize blood sugar and energy levels and is involved in everything from making enzymes to keeping our immune system in good working order. Given all this, it's no wonder protein takes the spotlight whenever menopause and nutrition come up in conversation. As important as protein is, putting it on a pedestal will make it more difficult to find balance.

WHY PROTEIN IS A KEY INGREDIENT IN MENOPAUSE

- Although there are no specific protein guidelines for menopause, a modest increase in protein intake (1.0 to 1.2 g/kg body weight) may help counteract the hormonal and age-related changes that affect muscle mass, bone health, and metabolism.
- Our brain uses the amino acids from protein to make neurotransmitters that influence mood, memory, and motivation—all of which can be challenging in midlife.
- Protein enhances satiety and helps balance blood sugar.
- Foods that are rich in protein are usually nutrient dense and good sources of iron, vitamin B_{12}, zinc, and magnesium.

Many women I speak with worry they're not eating enough protein and are confused about how much to eat, along with when and what types are best. Protein requirements are individual and can vary with height, bone structure, and activity level. If only it were as easy as looking it up in a chart!

The Power of Protein

Protein is a building block for strength, structure, and hormones. But it also influences our mood and energy on a daily basis. Let's take a closer look at its role in menopause.

Building and Maintaining Muscle

Muscle does much more than make us strong; it makes us more resilient to the impact of the hormonal changes of menopause on our body, especially those that increase our risk of osteoporosis and heart disease. Maintaining muscle is also one of the most tangible ways to age well. In the Women's Health Initiative (WHI) study, a higher protein intake (1.2 g/kg body weight) was associated with a 32 percent lower risk of frailty and better physical function.[8] Muscle mass and strength training are linked to better cognitive health, too. Most importantly, muscle helps us feel strong and confident *in* our bodies.

As we age, it's not as easy to build and maintain muscle. As estrogen levels decline during menopause, it can affect muscle strength and function. Our body also doesn't use protein as efficiently as it once did, so we may need to eat a little more to compensate, which is why protein is a key ingredient. There are two things needed to build muscle in menopause:

- Adequate amounts of protein, overall and on a per-meal basis
- Adequate mechanical stress to the muscles through strength training

Strength training, or resistance training, is all about building muscle strength and endurance by working against resistance, like your body weight, dumbbells, resistance bands, or machines. If you're new, start with the basics—think squats, lunges, push-ups, and rows—using just your body weight or light weights or even soup cans! As you gain experience, you can move on to more complex movements and heavier weights. Aim for two to three sessions a week, covering all major muscle groups and remember that consistency is key. It's never too late to start, and if you're uncertain about form or technique, working with a certified trainer can be a great help.

Maintaining Bone Health

Along with muscle, adequate protein intake is also an important determinant of bone health. People with higher muscle mass tend to have increased bone mass. Since one-third of bone mass is made of protein, it's easy to see why protein in our diet can help our bones stay strong in menopause. But adequacy, not excess, is the key word here, as most studies looking at protein and bone density have failed to find benefits at high intakes.

Feeling Full and Satisfied

When we connect and stay focused on how our food makes us feel, it will become much easier, and intuitive, to choose these nourishing foods more often. Protein helps us feel full and satisfied because it takes longer to digest, prolonging the feeling of fullness. Together with carbohydrates, protein also helps to reduce ghrelin and increase leptin, two of the hormones involved in appetite regulation.

> ## Satiation versus Satiety
>
> It's a common misconception that the words *satiation* and *satiety* are synonyms, but in fact, each refers to a distinct state. Satiation refers to the feeling of fullness and satisfaction during a meal. In other words, it's the point at which we've eaten enough to feel full. It is influenced by various factors, including the balance of protein, carbohydrates, and fats in the meal. Satiety refers to the feeling of fullness and lack of hunger between meals. It helps regulate our overall food intake and influences our eating patterns over time. Appetite hormones such as ghrelin, leptin, and GLP-1 play important roles in satiety.

The Recipe for Adding More Protein to Your Plate

When it comes to protein, quality and quantity are equally important. Understanding both will help you build balanced, nourishing meals with confidence—no counting grams or carrying food scales needed.

Understand Protein Quality

Protein quality impacts how effectively our bodies can use the protein we eat. A complete protein has all nine essential amino acids our bodies need but can't make on their own. You'll find these mostly in animal products like meat, dairy, and eggs, but a few plants like quinoa and soy have them, too, which is why soy is a key ingredient. On the other hand, incomplete proteins are missing one or more of these amino acids and are common in things like grains, nuts, and beans. The good news is you can mix and match these incomplete proteins, like pairing beans with rice, to get all the amino acids you need.

A key player in this process might be the amino acid leucine, an essential amino acid that triggers muscle protein synthesis. This leucine trigger may be more important in helping older adults maintain and build muscle mass, which can be made even more challenging in menopause because of hormonal changes. Eating foods with sufficient leucine is one of the ways to support building and maintaining muscle in midlife. Most animal sources of protein are good sources of leucine. Soy foods, owing to soy's status as a complete protein, are equally rich in leucine. For example, 1 cup (160 g) edamame provides 2 g of leucine, which is on par with 3 ounces (85 g) of meat.

Understand Serving Sizes

If we assume that one of our goals is to build muscle and strength, then aiming for about 25 g of protein per meal is enough to stimulate muscle protein synthesis (MPS) in most people, including older adults.[9] Instead of counting grams of protein at every meal, or carrying around a kitchen scale in your bag, here's how I estimate protein. Knowing this will boost your confidence that you're getting enough.

First, think of a Broadway production, or even a child's school play. Most will feature a main character (or two) and several supporting roles. If we apply these roles to protein, we get something that looks like this:

Main character: 15 to 25 g per serving

Supporting role: 5 to 15 g per serving

If you build a meal with one or two main characters, you can be confident that you have enough protein for that meal to be satisfying and nourishing. Think of a chicken breast, ¾ cup (175 g) of Greek yogurt, or ¾ cup (120 g) of edamame. Many of the foods that can provide main character protein are either animal or soy based, so you get the bonus of knowing that these are complete proteins.

If you choose several supporting roles, like egg, hummus, or cheese, you can easily get the same amount of protein as a starring role. Many of these will also be complete proteins, and if they aren't, you don't have to worry as these foods aren't usually eaten on their own but with a grain. Hummus, for example, is often eaten with pita bread, and the combination of amino acids from chickpeas and wheat complement each other. The same is true if you choose several smaller cast members like nuts, seeds, and nut butter. The key take-home message here isn't to choose the starring roles all the time but to know how to mix and match the roles so that your play is a success.

PROTEIN AT A GLANCE: ESTIMATING HOW MUCH IS ON YOUR PLATE

Main Characters (15 g+)	Protein (g)	Supporting Characters (5–15 g)	Protein (g)
Chicken breast (3½ ounces/100 g)	32	Beans and lentils (½ cup/95 g)	8–19
Tuna, canned (5 ounces/142 g)	28	Cottage cheese (½ cup/105 g)	13
Turkey breast (3½ ounces/100 g)	26	Eggs (2)	12
Seitan (3½ ounces/100 g)	25	Pumpkin seeds (¼ cup/30 g)	9
Salmon (3½ ounces/100 g)	24	Peanut butter (2 tablespoons)	7
Cooked shrimp (3½ ounces/100 g)	24	Cow milk (1 cup/240 ml)	9
Lean beef (3½ ounces/100 g)	21	Whole wheat pasta, cooked (1 cup/140 g)	8.5
Tempeh (3½ ounces/100 g)	19.9	Almonds (¼ cup/35 g)	8
Edamame (1 cup/160 g)	18.5	Soy milk (1 cup/240 ml)	7
Tofu (3½ ounces/100 g)	18	Whole grain bread (2 slices)	6–8
Greek yogurt (¾ cup/175 g)	17.5	Hemp seeds (2 tablespoons)	6

Key Ingredient: Fiber

You know you're in midlife when you choose your cereal for the fiber instead of the toy. All kidding aside, fiber is a regular topic of conversation in midlife because fiber is a key ingredient, and chances are you're not getting enough of it. Surveys regularly find that as many as 95 percent of Americans aren't getting the recommended amounts of 25 to 39 g per day, and that women are only getting 13.5 g on average.[10] Trust me when I tell you that adding more fiber to your plate is one of the best investments you can make for menopause and your health in general, as studies show that eating enough fiber can reduce your risk of death from all causes by 15 to 30 percent.[11]

WHY FIBER IS A KEY INGREDIENT IN MENOPAUSE

- Fiber supports cardiovascular health by lowering cholesterol and blood sugar. Including 10 g of soluble fiber every day can reduce cholesterol levels by up to 10 percent and reduce HbA1c (a blood test that shows a 3-month average of blood sugar levels) levels by 0.5 to 1 percent.[12]
- High-fiber diets are associated with fewer menopausal symptoms, including hot flashes and sleep disturbances.[13]
- Eating enough fiber helps prevent constipation, which reduces the risk of pelvic floor problems that are more common in menopause, including prolapse.
- High-fiber diets have been shown to reduce several cancers, including breast and colon cancer. It's estimated that every 10 g of added fiber can reduce colon cancer risk by around 7 percent.[14]
- Fiber supports the health of our microbiome by keeping our gut bacteria well fed. This promotes digestive health and may reduce symptoms such as bloating, diarrhea, and constipation.
- Fiber-rich foods help promote satiety and fullness (page 98).

Types of Fiber

Fiber is a type of starchy carbohydrate that humans can't digest. The two main types of fiber are insoluble and soluble. Fibers can also be categorized based on their viscosity (ability to form a gel-like substance) and ability to be fermented by gut bacteria, each providing different health benefits. Think of insoluble fiber as a pipe cleaner and soluble fiber as a sponge. Both are important and can support our health in different ways. One of the reasons I don't recommend low-carbohydrate diets is that they eliminate the most convenient and delicious sources of fiber—fruits and whole grains.

Soluble Fiber

Soluble fiber is viscous and acts like a gel as it passes through our digestive tract, soaking things up along the way. This is how soluble fiber, like the type found in oatmeal, helps reduce cholesterol. Beta-glucan is a special type of soluble fiber found in whole grains such as oatmeal, oat bran, barley, mushrooms, and even some seaweeds. The versatility of its sources means there are plenty of ways to add it to your daily plate, either in a bowl of oatmeal in the morning or a stir-fry with mushrooms for dinner. You'll want to aim for 3 g of beta-glucan per day if you're trying to reduce your cholesterol, although some studies have found that 1.5 g per day, the amount found in 1 cup (235 g) of cooked oatmeal, was just as effective.[15]

Insoluble Fiber

Insoluble fiber does not dissolve in water and, as such, adds bulk to our stool and helps keep things regular. You'll find this type of fiber in many foods, including whole grains and fruits with edible skins. Because of insoluble fiber's pipe cleaner effect, some people are sensitive to large amounts and benefit from a gradual increase of high-fiber foods to their usual diets. See page 99 for tips on easing the transition to a high-fiber diet.

The Recipe for Adding More Fiber to Your Plate

Many people struggle to meet their daily fiber goals or feel like they need to always choose the highest-fiber food, which can lead to boredom and mealtime blahs. It's easy to give your fiber intake a boost with a plant-forward mindset and the following tips.

Eat More Plants

All plants are sources of fiber, so you can keep your fiber goals intuitive by keeping this in mind. Whether you're having soup, a sandwich, or a snack, get in the habit of asking yourself, "Can I add a plant here?" Allow yourself to lower the bar when it comes to serving sizes, too; every little bit adds up, and it all counts.

Front-Load the Day

Breakfast isn't necessarily the most important meal of the day, but it can be the easiest way to include more fiber. Oats can be made overnight or cooked quickly on the stove in the morning. Fruit smoothies are another quick meal that can include fresh or frozen fruit for a satisfying high-fiber start to the morning. Try the Key Lime Overnight Oats (page 115) or the Blueberry Banana Tofu Smoothie (page 234) if you're looking for ideas.

Include Beans and Lentils More Often

You'll find a minimum of 8 to 10 g of fiber in every 1 cup (190 g) cooked serving of most beans and lentils. Keep your pantry stocked with canned chickpeas, black beans, and lentils and store shelled edamame in the freezer. Delicious dishes that feature meat and beans, like the Tortilla Soup (page 144), show how easy it is to add more plants to your plate.

Snack on Nuts and Seeds

Most nuts and seeds provide 1 to 3 g of fiber per ounce, making them an ideal topper for things like salads and yogurt and the perfect crunchy sidekick to almost any snack. It's easy to keep mixed nuts handy at home or on the go. Try the Crunchy Miso Snack and Salad Topper (page 208) for a perfect hit of satisfying crunch.

Don't Fear Fruit

Once known as nature's perfect snack, fruit's reputation took a hit when the low-carb and keto crazes went mainstream. Many people ask me whether fruits are too high in sugar to be enjoyed regularly and are relieved when I tell them the short answer is no. Fruits' sugars are well balanced by the fiber they provide, and there's ample evidence to show that eating fruit every day is associated with living a longer, healthier life.[16]

FIBER-FRIENDLY FOODS		
FOOD	**Total Fiber (g) per Serving**	**Soluble Fiber (g) per Serving**
Legumes		
Black beans, cooked (1 cup/170 g)	13.0	2.4
Chickpeas, cooked (1 cup/200 g)	10.3	2.5
Edamame, cooked (1 cup/160 g)	8.1	3.0
Lentils, cooked (1 cup/190 g)	10.5	1.2
Grains		
Barley, cooked (1 cup/160 g)	6.0	1.6
Oats, cooked (1 cup/235 g)	5.5	1.5
Popcorn, air-popped (3 cups/30 g)	3.5	-
Quinoa, cooked (¾ cup/140 g)	5.2	0.9
Fruits		
Apples with skin (1 medium)	4.4	1.0
Avocado (½ fruit)	6.7	2.1
Figs, dried (¼ cup/40 g)	3.9	1.9
Pear with skin (1 medium)	5.5	1.2
Raspberries (1 cup/120 g)	8.0	1.8
Vegetables		
Broccoli, cooked (½ cup/80 g)	2.4	1.2
Brussels sprouts, cooked (½ cup/80 g)	3.8	2.0
Green peas, cooked (½ cup/75 g)	4.3	1.3
Sweet potato, cooked (1 medium)	3.9	1.8
Other		
Almonds (¼ cup/35 g)	3.8	0.5
Chia seeds (2 tablespoons)	9.6	1.0
Flax, ground (2 tablespoons)	3.8	1.3

Tips for a Smooth Transition to a High-Fiber Diet

The most frequent fiber complaint I hear from people is that it makes them bloated and gassy. This is especially true with beans, lentils, and some cruciferous vegetables like Brussels sprouts and cauliflower. These foods contain raffinose, a type of carbohydrate we can't digest because we lack the enzyme alpha-galactosidase. Even though gas production is a good sign that your gut bacteria are enjoying a feast, so to speak, it can present a challenge. The problem usually arises when we add too much fiber too quickly, not giving our gut bacteria enough time to adjust. Here are some easy-to-digest tips:

- Cooked vegetables are easier to digest than raw (insoluble fiber is partially broken down with cooking).
- Start with beans and lentils that are naturally lower in raffinose, the gas-producing starch. Chickpeas, lentils (green, red, and brown), and black-eyed peas are good ones to try. Black beans and kidney beans are known to be gassier, so keep that in mind if you're new to eating beans. Start with small amounts and increase slowly. Add 1 to 2 tablespoons of beans to a salad or start with hummus and crackers as a snack a few times a week.
- If using dried beans, allow at least twelve hours to soak the beans overnight before cooking them in fresh water. This cuts down the amount of gas-producing oligosaccharides (such as raffinose) significantly, as does the cooking and canning process with canned beans.
- When eating beans and lentils, consider using a common over-the-counter enzyme supplement that contains alpha-galactosidase, such as Beano.

SUPPLEMENT:

Fiber

Fiber supplements can be a convenient way to add fiber to your diet, but not all fiber supplements are created equally. Knowing what problem you're trying to solve will determine which type of fiber will work best for the job.

HOW TO CHOOSE THE BEST FIBER SUPPLEMENT			
Type of Fiber Supplement	**Best Uses**	**Look For**	**Watch For**
Psyllium	Digestive symptoms (e.g., diarrhea, constipation), cholesterol lowering, blood sugar stabilization	Whole psyllium husk, or psyllium fiber in powder or capsule form	Can cause bloating or gas in sensitive individuals
Methylcellulose	Constipation	Methylcellulose powder, often in Citrucel	Less likely to cause gas but can cause bloating in large amounts
Wheat Dextrin	General fiber boost, mild constipation	Soluble fiber supplements like Benefiber (US only)	May not be effective for constipation in some individuals
Inulin	Gut microbiome support, prebiotic	Inulin in powder or supplement form, often from chicory root	Can cause gas and bloating in some people, especially those with IBS
Acacia Fiber	Gut microbiome support, gentle on digestion	Acacia fiber powder, often labeled as gentle fiber	Generally well tolerated but may cause mild digestive discomfort

Key Ingredient: Calcium

Calcium is the most abundant mineral in the human body, and 99 percent of the calcium in our body is found in our bones. Many women I talk to have a bottle of calcium supplements sitting on a shelf at the back of a cupboard, but most are confused about how much calcium they need and whether supplements are even necessary. Let's dive into why calcium's spot on our key ingredient list is well deserved.

WHY CALCIUM IS A KEY INGREDIENT IN MENOPAUSE

- Calcium strengthens bones and helps muscles contract and relax, including the heart.
- Our body carefully regulates calcium levels, using bone reserves when dietary intake is low.
- Low calcium intake may lead to sleep issues, particularly trouble falling asleep and poor sleep quality.[17]
- Higher calcium intake is linked to a lower risk of colon cancer.

A Closer Look at Calcium

Our bodies rely on calcium being available when needed, and our bones act like a bank, allowing a withdrawal of calcium to be made if our dietary calcium intake is low. If we're getting enough calcium from food (or supplements), the balance in our bones is topped up. If not, the withdrawals continue, increasing the risk of osteopenia and osteoporosis. If you're wondering how your current calcium intake measures up, I've included information about online calcium calculators in the resources section on page 255.

To Supplement or Not to Supplement

When I first started practicing, it was a no-brainer to tell women to eat two to three servings of calcium-rich foods per day and that taking a calcium supplement was good insurance to meet the recommended target of 1,200 mg per day. At the time, it was generally accepted that more calcium was better than less—and this was especially true for people over forty. I received the same advice from my doctor when we realized I was on track for early menopause.

This advice was given with one goal in mind—to reduce the risk of developing osteoporosis and, more importantly, fractures. Fractures are no joke, with an estimated one in three women and one in five men suffering an osteoporotic fracture during their lifetime. And since it was (and still is) well known that calcium is critical for *building* healthy bone, it was assumed that it also helped *maintain* healthy bone. However, research in the mid-2000s started to take a closer look at whether calcium supplements prevented fractures. To many people's surprise, they probably don't. Even I was surprised when a meta-analysis concluded that the use of supplements that included calcium, vitamin D, or both was not associated with a lower risk of fractures when compared with placebo or no treatment.[18]

When this news made headlines, many people misinterpreted the findings and made the mistake of equating dietary calcium with calcium supplements. To be clear, the recommendation to get enough calcium still stands—preferably using a food-first approach.

Not All Calcium Is Created Equally

The top calcium-containing foods include dairy products (milk, yogurt, and cheese), leafy green vegetables (kale, collard greens, and bok choy), canned fish with bones (sardines and salmon), nuts and seeds (almonds, sesame seeds, and chia seeds), and legumes (soybeans and white beans). Calcium recommendations assume that you'll be getting calcium from a variety of foods, some of which will be better absorbed than others. The bioavailability, which is the amount that is actually absorbed and used by your body, is not the same for all foods. Factors such as the food's composition, presence of inhibitors like oxalates (compounds in leafy greens) and phytates (found in seeds and grains), and how the food is prepared can all influence calcium absorption. For example:

- A cup (240 ml) of milk contains around 300 mg of calcium, with a bioavailability of about 30 percent. So, about 100 mg of calcium is absorbed from a cup of milk.
- Leafy greens, on the other hand, often boast a calcium bioavailability of 50 percent or more but provide fewer milligrams of calcium per serving, meaning much larger amounts may be needed.[19] Keep in mind that cooked leafy greens have more easily absorbed calcium.
- The amount of bioavailable calcium in a cup (240 ml) of milk is equal to that in 3 cups (480 g) of cooked broccoli, 2 cups (130 g) of raw kale, or ¾ cup (105 g) of almonds.

CALCIUM CONTENT OF COMMON FOODS	
FOOD	**Total Calcium (mg) per Serving**
Tofu, firm (½ cup/125 g)	434
Sardines, canned (3.75 ounces/106 g)	350
Yogurt (¾ cup/175 g)	332
Cheddar cheese (1½ oz/40 g)	307
Milk, low-fat, skim, whole (1 cup/240 ml)	300
Collard greens, cooked (1 cup/190 g)	268
Molasses (1 tablespoon)	190
Chia seeds (2 tablespoons)	179
Edamame, cooked (1 cup/160 g)	170
White beans (1 cup/180 g)	161
Figs, dried (8 figs)	135
Almonds (1 ounce/30 g)	75

Calcium Is Better with Friends

You've probably heard that calcium, magnesium, and vitamin D are all involved in bone health. Magnesium helps activate vitamin D, which in turn helps increase calcium absorption. One of the reasons a plant-forward pattern of eating is beneficial in menopause is because beans, lentils, nuts, and seeds are excellent sources of magnesium. Leafy greens also contain vitamin K, which is converted to vitamin K_2 by gut bacteria. Vitamin K_2 is also involved in helping calcium get into our bones, but exactly how much we need isn't known yet.

Vitamin D is actually a hormone and can be made when our skin is exposed to sun. Even though we can make and store quite a bit of vitamin D during the summer months, you may still need a supplement as there are only a handful of foods that provide vitamin D. You'll find decent amounts in salmon and tuna, as well as fortified dairy and nondairy beverages. Try the Sweet Potato Salmon Cakes (page 179) for a delicious way to include more calcium and vitamin D.

SUPPLEMENT: Calcium

Although most people can get enough calcium from their diet, some may still choose to supplement. If you decide to go that route, keep these tips in mind:

- **The type:** Most calcium supplements contain either calcium carbonate or calcium citrate. Calcium carbonate is the most common, owing largely to its affordability, but calcium citrate may have a slight advantage because it doesn't require an acidic environment to be absorbed. In general, absorption of calcium supplements is enhanced when taken with a meal.
- **The dose:** Most calcium supplements come in doses ranging from 100 to 500 mg, but it's important to know that the absorption of calcium decreases when more than 500 mg is ingested at one time.
- **Side effects and interactions:** Constipation is a common side effect of calcium supplements, and there may be interactions with common prescription medications to consider, including thyroid and blood pressure medications. Talk to your doctor or pharmacist before starting any supplement.

The Recipe for Adding More Calcium to Your Plate

Prioritize satisfaction over nutrition*ism*. Meaning don't rely solely on the calcium content of a food to decide what you should eat. Here are some tips for choosing calcium-rich foods intuitively and with intention.

Include Dairy

Foods such as milk, yogurt, and cheese always top the list of calcium-rich foods for good reason: They provide a substantial amount of calcium per serving and often vitamin D and protein as well. We know that protein intake also influences bone strength, and getting calcium, protein, and vitamin D in one place is undeniably convenient. If you enjoy and tolerate dairy, add it to the plate!

Plan for Density and Diversity

There's no shortage of nondairy sources of calcium. Most nondairy milk beverages are fortified with it. For example, you can use fortified soy milk in a smoothie to benefit from phytoestrogens, calcium, and vitamin D. Firm or extra-firm tofu is another great nondairy source as long as it's "calcium set," meaning that calcium has been added to the process. If calcium sulphate is listed as one of the ingredients, you can count on it providing about 200 mg of calcium per ⅓ cup (85 g).

A 3.75 ounce (106 g) can of sardines provides 350 mg, while a 5-ounce can (142 g) of salmon also provides 350 mg of calcium. Why canned? Because of the bones, which are not removed before canning and are soft and barely noticeable by the time you crack open the tin.

Cook Your Greens

Low-oxalate greens including kale, broccoli, and bok choy will provide more bioavailable calcium than greens such as Swiss chard and spinach. Cooking your greens will help reduce the oxalate content and increase the amount of calcium you can absorb. For example, 1 cup (180 g) of cooked spinach has 245 mg of calcium while 1 cup (30 g) of raw spinach has only 30 mg.

Undiet It! The Myth of Best Foods

Are you making mental notes of which foods are "best"? Watch for that sneaky all-or-nothing mindset. I'm not saying you should *never* eat a spinach salad or *always* choose broccoli. Choose what you enjoy and is accessible to you and use this information to help guide your choices. Remember, diversity is the name of the game when it comes to nutrition.

Key Ingredient: Omega-3 Fatty Acids

Omega-3 and omega-6 fats are polyunsaturated fatty acids, sometimes referred to as PUFAs. They are described as essential because the human body can't make them—which means we need to get them from food or supplements. Unlike omega-3s, which are found in only a few foods, omega-6s are widely available in many foods and most people easily get enough of them through food.

WHY OMEGA-3S ARE A KEY INGREDIENT IN MENOPAUSE

- The omega-3 fatty acids eicosapentaenoic acid (EPA) and docosahexaenoic acid (DHA) can help keep your heart healthy by lowering triglyceride levels by 15 to 25 percent[20] and may also help lower blood pressure.[21]
- DHA is the main fatty acid in the brain and helps keep your brain healthy and sharp. Research also shows that eating these fats regularly might help lower the chances of depression and anxiety, which are both common during menopause.
- Omega-3s help calm inflammation in the body by reducing the production of substances like eicosanoids and cytokines, which are linked to inflammation.
- There's some limited evidence that omega-3s may help to lessen the frequency and intensity of hot flashes and aid in improving sleep patterns.
- Omega-3s may also play a protective role in bone health, along with vitamin D and calcium.

Types of Omega-3 Fatty Acids

The three main types of omega-3 fatty acids are EPA, DHA, and alpha-linolenic acid (ALA). However, not all omega-3s are created equally, and understanding the differences among them is important.

EPA and DHA

EPA and DHA are found primarily in fish and can be used as is by the body when eaten. Although there is no specific recommended dietary allowance (RDA) for EPA and DHA, adults should aim for a combined average of 250 to 500 mg of EPA and DHA per day by eating two to three servings of fatty fish per week. The American Heart Association has suggested amounts up to 1,000 mg per day for individuals with existing heart disease.

ALA

ALA comes primarily from plants and is found in foods like flax, chia seeds, and walnuts. The recommended intake for adult women is 1.1 g per day. ALA can be converted into small amounts of EPA and DHA, but it's not a very efficient process.[22] This is why people who don't eat fish (for whatever reason) may choose to take a fish oil supplement or marine algae, which provides plant-based DHA.

The Recipe for Adding More Omega-3s to Your Plate

Getting enough omega-3s doesn't have to be complicated or require fancy cooking skills. Fish can be surprisingly simple to prepare, whether you're grilling, baking, or even just adding a can of sardines or salmon to a salad. Plant-based sources, like flax, chia seeds, and walnuts, may seem small, but those little additions add up.

Find Convenience in a Can

Fish, especially cold-water oily fish, such as salmon, mackerel, and sardines, are the most concentrated food sources of EPA and DHA. But buying and cooking fresh fish isn't always convenient, so keep tuna, salmon, and sardines in your pantry. Try the Tuna Salad with Cranberry (page 204) or the Sweet Potato Salmon Cakes (page 179), and you'll see how helpful the canned foods can be.

Canned fish is one of the most polarizing foods—people either love it or hate it. Many worry that this preserved fish is less healthy, but the nutrient content is on par with fresh fish. And some research has found that as consumption of canned fish goes up, the risk of colorectal cancer goes down, likely because including more fish from any source may reduce the risk of many cancers.[23]

The question of safety and sustainability remains top of mind for some people, including me. Heavy metals, such as mercury and cadmium, are more likely to be found in larger fish species, such as albacore and bluefin tuna. Reassuringly, most research has found that nonpregnant adults can safely eat canned tuna two to three times a week without concern. If sustainable fish is a priority, look for logos from the Marine Stewardship Council (MSC),

Aquaculture Stewardship Council (ASC), or Best Aquaculture Practices (BAP). These not-for-profit organizations certify that the seafood comes from a sustainable source.

Put the Shine on Shellfish

Don't let finned fish steal the spotlight. Shellfish like mussels, oysters, and shrimp can also be excellent sources of omega-3s and are great for putting variety on the menu. Try the shrimp variation of the Marinated Tofu and Soba Noodles with Bok Choy (page 183) if you're looking to switch things up.

Sprinkle Plant Sources into Your Day-to-Day

Plant-based sources of omega-3s, such as flax, chia seeds, and walnuts, may lack the potency of their fishy counterparts, but they're easy and convenient sources of ALA that deserve a place on your plate. For example, adding 1 tablespoon each of ground flax, chia seeds, and walnuts to your breakfast adds 3,500 mg of ALA in addition to the fiber, protein, and satisfaction they provide. For example, here's how you might estimate how much EPA and DHA could be made from 3,500 mg of ALA:

- EPA: 3,500 mg of ALA × 5% to 10% conversion = 175 to 350 mg of EPA
- DHA: 3,500 mg of ALA × 2% to 5% conversion = 70 to 175 mg of DHA

As you can see, plant sources of omega-3 fatty acids can still make a sizable dent in meeting our needs. Try the Baked Chocolate Chip Oatmeal (page 121), Very Berry Chia Jam (page 125), and Miso Flax Crackers (page 212).

Cook with Care

As with all fats, the time, temperature, and cooking method can impact the quantity and stability of essential fatty acids. Baking and steaming fish appear to better preserve the omega-3 content than grilling and frying at high temperatures. Similarly, flaxseed oil is highly sensitive to heat and should not be used for cooking at high temperatures. Baking with ground flax is fine at temperatures up to 350°F (175°C).

SUPPLEMENT:
Omega-3 Supplements

Not everyone loves the taste of fish. If that's you, fish oil supplements can be a helpful tool in meeting your omega-3 requirements. Before taking a fish oil supplement, it's important to note that it can interact with blood thinners, blood pressure medication, and chemotherapy (and should be avoided if you have a shellfish allergy, since the risk of cross contamination is high). In other words, talk to a health-care professional before taking them. Here are some other things to consider when looking at supplements:

- Supplements containing EPA and DHA can come from a variety of fish and seafood including salmon, mackerel, herring, and krill. While many claims are made about which is best, there's no clear winner in my opinion.
- Vegans and vegetarians may want to look at microalgae supplements, which can provide up to 250 mg of DHA from a nonanimal source.
- Fish oil supplements come in two forms: triglycerides (TG) and ethyl esters (EE). The triglyceride form is the natural fat found in fish and is similar to the fats we usually eat, which makes it easier for the body to absorb. The ethyl ester form is synthetic and allows for higher concentrations of EPA and DHA, but it might not absorb as well as triglycerides. So, you might need higher doses to get the same benefits.
- Fish burps are the most common side effect of omega-3 supplements. The best tip for reducing this is to take your supplements with a meal earlier in the day; you can also try keeping the capsules in the freezer. Lowering the temperature of the oil in the capsules makes them more viscous and less likely to repeat on you as oils at room temperature.

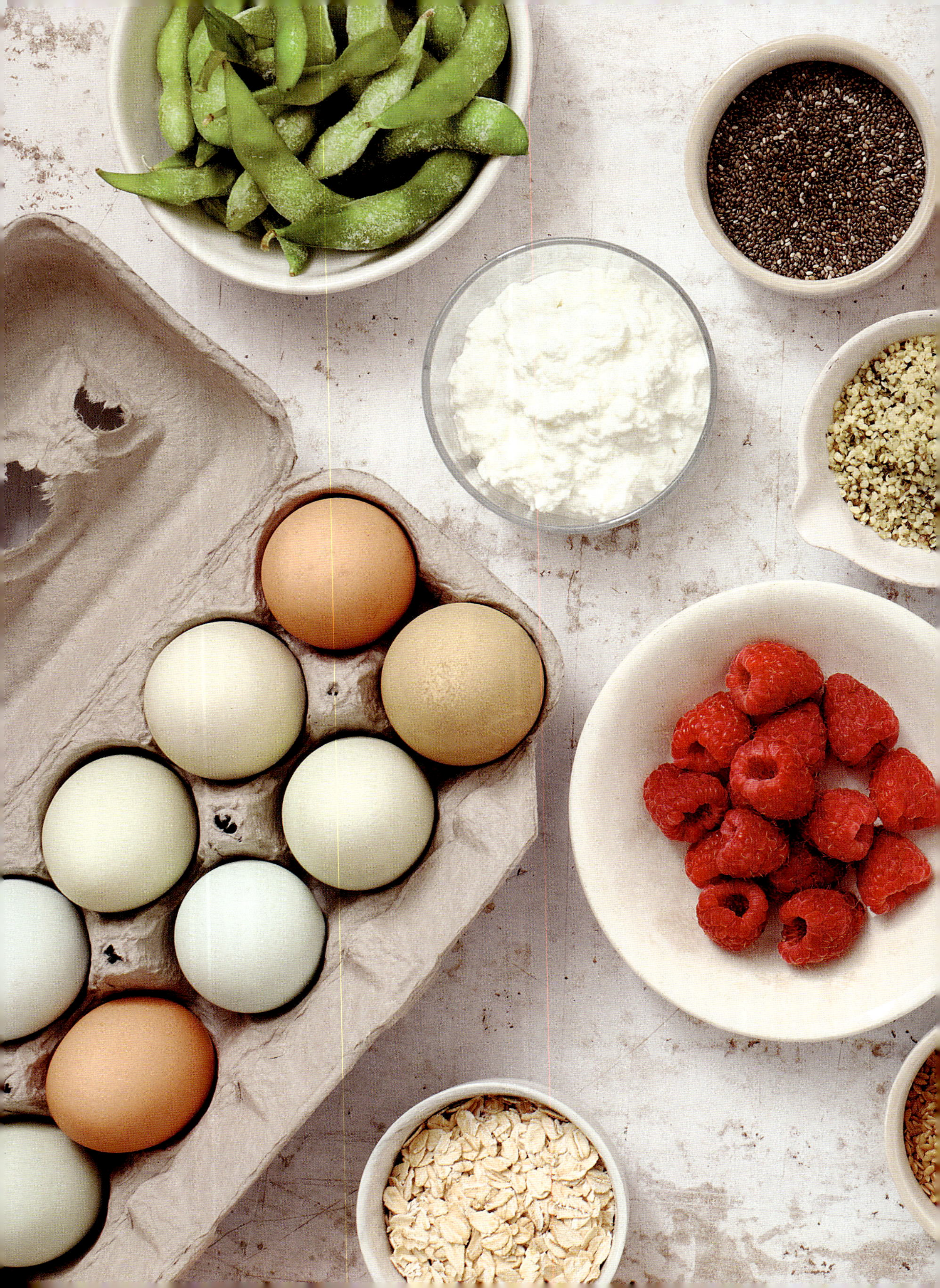

PART 4

The Recipes

Breakfast All Day

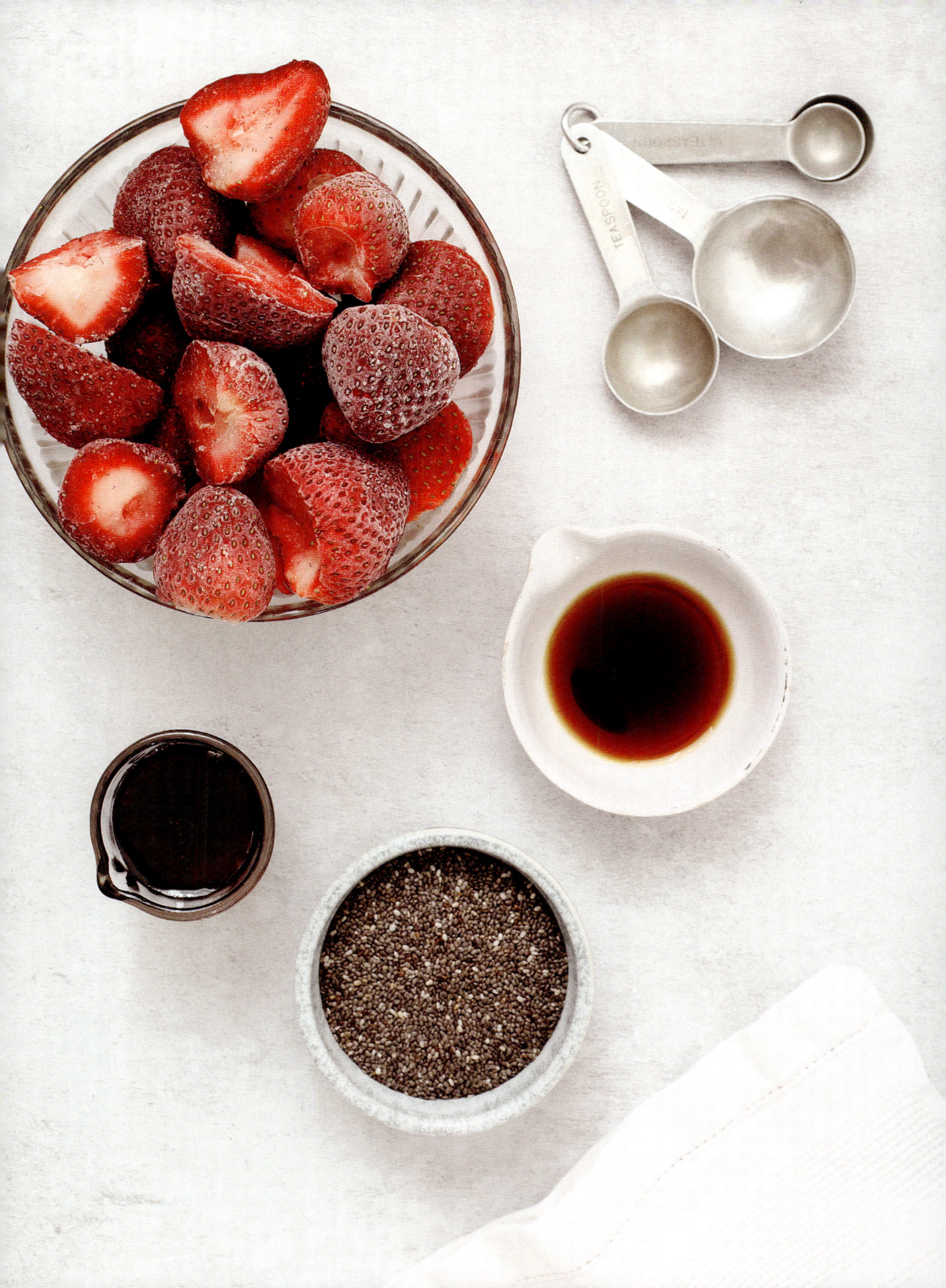
TEASPOON

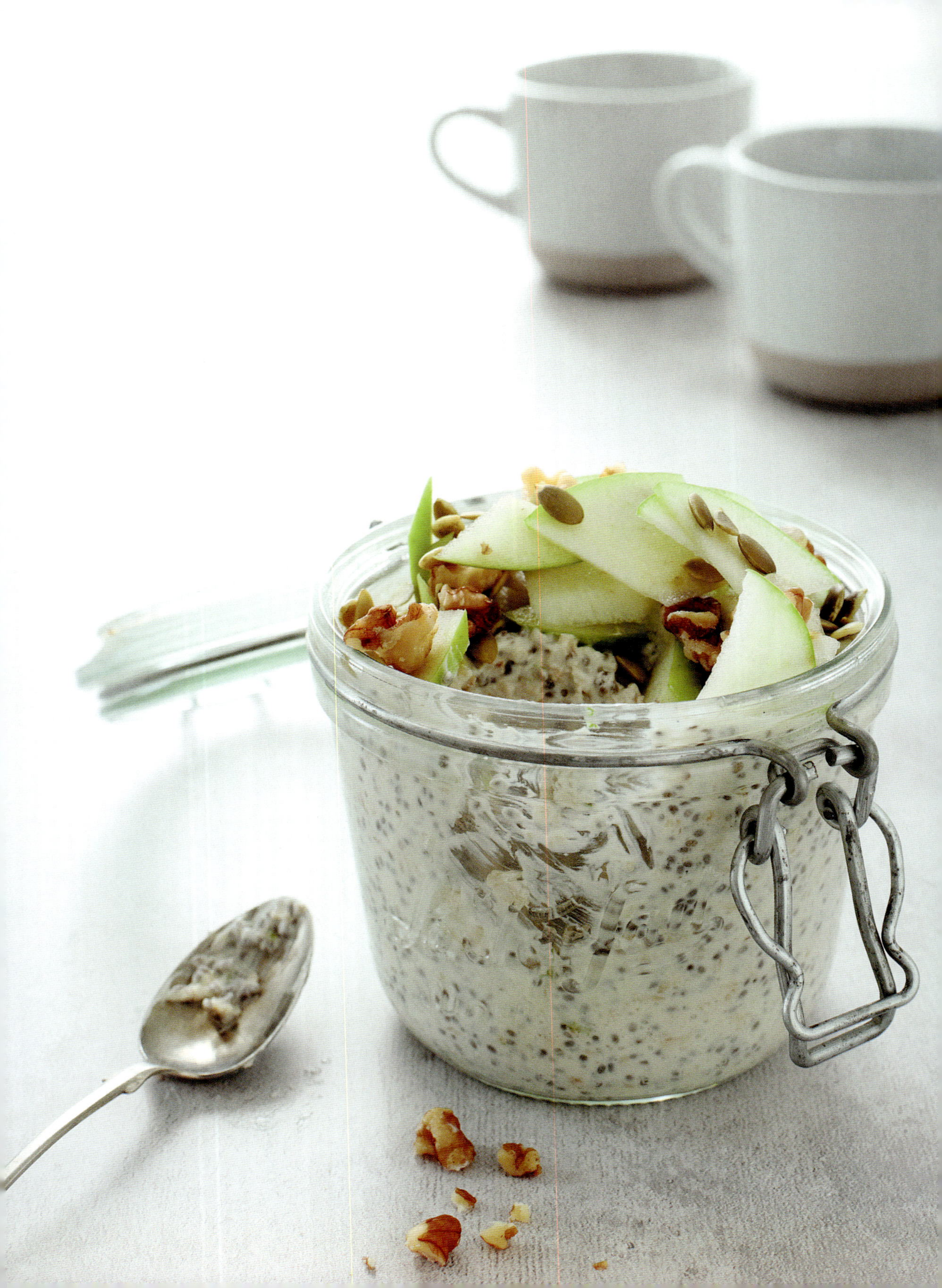

Key Lime Overnight Oats

+ **SOY & PHYTOESTROGENS** + **PROTEIN** + **FIBER** + **CALCIUM** + **OMEGA-3**

Makes 2 servings

Oats deserve a spot at the breakfast table, but many people avoid them because they take too long to prepare or are seen as too high in carbohydrates. Overnight oats solve both problems, offering a make-ahead option packed with beta-glucan, a type of soluble fiber that supports healthy cholesterol and blood sugar levels. This fresh take on oatmeal will keep you full and satisfied all morning. While any milk works, soy milk's mild nutty flavor and hot-flash-fighting phytoestrogens make it an easy choice.

---

1 cup (240 ml) soy milk

⅔ cup (155 g) vanilla Greek yogurt

Zest and juice of 1 lime

2 tablespoons maple syrup

1 cup (100 g) rolled oats

2 tablespoons chia seeds

Fresh fruit, flax, nuts, or seeds, for topping (optional)

---

1 Place the soy milk, yogurt, lime juice, and the maple syrup in a 2-cup (475 ml) jar or container with a lid.

2 Stir well to combine, then add the rolled oats, chia seeds, and lime zest. Stir well, cover, and refrigerate overnight or for a minimum of 6 hours.

3 Before serving, add the toppings of your choice for extra texture and satisfaction, if desired. Refrigerate any unused portions and use within three days.

Note: The minor differences in the amount of protein and fiber between steel-cut and rolled oats (see "Understanding Oats" box page 116) aren't enough to make one a better choice than the other. Lead with satisfaction and choose the type of oats you enjoy!

In a hurry? Turn this overnight oat recipe into quick oats by heating the oats, chia seeds, and soy milk in the microwave on high for 60 to 90 seconds. Once heated, mix in the lime juice, lime zest, maple syrup, and yogurt.

Top up! Add fruit for a fiber boost. Adding ½ cup (60 g) of raspberries will add another 4 g of fiber to this already high-fiber breakfast.

UNDERSTANDING OATS

I often jokingly refer to myself as the chief defender of oats, jumping to oatmeal's defense whenever someone suggests that oats aren't healthy or are too high in carbs. Here is what you need to know before choosing your oats.

Rolled Oats (Old-Fashioned Oats): Cooking time = 4 to 5 minutes

- **What are they?** This is the most common type of oats you'll find. They're made by taking whole oat groats and flattening them between large rollers.
- **Preparation:** Rolled oats are incredibly versatile. You can cook them on the stovetop, microwave them, or even soak them overnight for a no-cook option. They absorb liquid well, making them perfect for creamy oatmeal.

Steel-Cut Oats: Cooking time = 20 to 30 minutes

- **What are they?** These oats are made from whole oat groats, just like rolled oats, but they're chopped into small pieces rather than flattened.
- **Preparation:** Steel-cut oats take longer to cook than rolled oats, but their nutty, chewy texture can be worth the wait, especially if you prefer a hearty porridge. Simmer them on the stovetop or soak overnight.

Quick Oats: Cooking time = 1 to 2 minutes

- **What are they?** Quick oats are essentially rolled oats that have been chopped into smaller pieces to reduce cooking time.
- **Preparation:** As the name suggests, they cook quickly and are great when you're in a rush.

Instant Oats: Cooking time = < 1 minute

- **What are they?** These are precooked and dried oats, often with added flavorings and toppings.
- **Preparation:** Just add hot water or microwave them, and they're ready in a jiffy. They're convenient and great when you don't have access to a stove or microwave as only hot water is required.

Carrot Cake Overnight Oats

+ SOY & PHYTOESTROGENS + PROTEIN + FIBER + CALCIUM

Makes 2 servings

There's something indulgent and comforting about starting the day with a breakfast that tastes like cake! I love this recipe because it balances the familiar texture of rolled oats with the satisfying power of soy milk, protein powder, and warming carrot cake spices. Designed to make mornings easier, this overnight recipe will be a welcome addition to your breakfast table.

---

1 cup (240 ml) soy milk

2 tablespoons coconut milk

1 teaspoon ground cinnamon

1 scoop (30 g) vanilla protein powder or ⅓ cup (80 g) vanilla Greek yogurt (see note)

½ teaspoon pure vanilla extract

¼ teaspoon ground ginger

Pinch of nutmeg

½ cup (50 g) rolled oats

1 medium carrot, peeled and grated

---

1 Whisk together the soy milk, coconut milk, cinnamon, protein powder, vanilla, ginger, and nutmeg in a medium bowl or dish (I use a 2-cup/475 ml mason jar).

2 Fold in the oats and carrot and refrigerate, covered, for at least 4 hours or overnight, until the oats are soft and creamy.

3 In the morning, stir, heat if desired by warming in a microwave for 60 to 90 seconds, and enjoy!

Note: Using Greek yogurt instead of protein powder results in a very similar taste and texture, with only a small reduction in overall protein content.

Undiet It! Protein Powder

People are often surprised to see an intuitive eating dietitian recommend protein powder, because of its association with diet culture, but I welcome this easy and satisfying addition to my own plate. Thanks to food neutrality, I'm not pulled into labeling foods as "good" or "bad," "healthy" or "unhealthy." I'm free to enjoy any food, including the ones that make my life easier, and protein powder does just that. Here's an at-a-glance guide to the types of protein powders available.

GUIDE TO PROTEIN POWDERS

Protein Powder Type	Source	Benefits	Best Uses
Whey	Milk	Complete protein, fast absorption, muscle recovery	Most versatile all-around protein, easiest to incorporate without affecting taste or texture
Casein	Milk	Complete protein, slow digestion, sustained release of amino acids	Good option when goals are satiety and satisfaction
Soy	Soybeans	Complete protein, heart health	Can help meet phytoestrogen and/or soy protein goals for cholesterol and heart health Note: Soy isolates undergo an extra step, resulting in slightly higher protein per serving and lower amounts of isoflavones.
Pea	Yellow peas	Hypoallergenic, contains iron	Good option for people who don't eat milk or soy, incomplete protein status can be overcome by choosing a mixed plant protein powder
Hemp	Hemp seeds	Complete protein, rich in omega-3s and omega-6s	Slightly lower in protein per serving, great way to top up protein in smoothies and baking

Tiramisu Overnight Oats

+ **SOY & PHYTOESTROGENS** + **PROTEIN** + **FIBER** + **CALCIUM** + **OMEGA-3**

Makes 2 servings

Coffee is a morning staple in many households. If you're like me, you may also find yourself with a small amount of leftover coffee some days, which is exactly what inspired this recipe. The richness of the brew pairs perfectly with the familiar flavors of cinnamon and vanilla in this overnight oatmeal. The soy milk and Greek yogurt provide extra creaminess in addition to protein, calcium, and phytoestrogens.

¾ cup (180 ml) soy milk

⅔ cup (65 g) rolled oats

⅓ cup (40 g) ground flax

½ cup (120 ml) brewed coffee of choice (including decaf), cooled

½ teaspoon pure vanilla extract

½ teaspoon ground cinnamon

Pinch of fine sea salt (optional)

¾ cup (175 g) plain Greek yogurt

Ground cinnamon and unsweetened cocoa powder, for garnish

---

1 Combine the soy milk, oats, flax, coffee, vanilla, cinnamon, and salt (if using) in a large jar or bowl. Cover and refrigerate for at least 4 hours or overnight, until the oats have absorbed the liquid.

2 The following day, evenly divide the oat mixture between two bowls or wide-mouthed glass jars, adding a layer of Greek yogurt in the center of each.

3 Sprinkle cinnamon and cocoa powder on top. Serve and enjoy!

Feast on This!

Coffee sometimes gets a bad rap, especially when it comes to health. But the evidence is pretty convincing that moderate coffee consumption (defined as less than 3 cups/700 ml per day) is associated with lower rates of many health conditions including type 2 diabetes, liver disease, and certain types of cancer. However, be aware that the type of coffee you drink may affect your cholesterol levels. Filtered coffee (using a paper filter) may be the better choice if you have high cholesterol, as unfiltered coffee contains the oils cafestol and kahweol, and can increase LDL, the so-called bad cholesterol that's associated with increasing your risk of heart disease. You might consider making this change if your cholesterol takes a jump in menopause.

Baked Chocolate Chip Oatmeal

+ **SOY & PHYTOESTROGENS** + **FIBER**

Makes 6 servings

Baked oatmeal is an easy and delicious alternative to warm, cooked oatmeal (porridge). It's firm and somewhat cake-like, with the added bonus that you can make it ahead of time. This basic recipe can be adapted to your taste by swapping the chocolate chips for ⅓ cup (40 g) of nuts, dried cranberries, or any other add-ins you enjoy. I often make this on Sunday evening to ensure a smooth start to the week. It also makes a great midday snack when you need a satisfying pick-me-up.

Extra virgin olive oil, for greasing the baking dish

3 medium ripe bananas, peeled

1 cup (240 ml) soy milk

1 teaspoon pure vanilla extract

1 large egg

2 cups (200 g) rolled oats

1½ teaspoons ground cinnamon

½ teaspoon baking soda

½ teaspoon fine sea salt

⅓ cup (40 g) ground flax

⅓ cup (60 g) chocolate chips

---

1 Preheat the oven to 375°F (190°C). Lightly grease a 9 × 9-inch (23 × 23 cm) baking dish with oil (or line it with parchment paper) and set aside.

2 Mash the bananas with a fork in a large bowl. Add the soy milk, vanilla, and egg and stir to combine.

3 Add the oats, cinnamon, baking soda, and salt to the banana mixture and stir until well combined, then fold in the flax and chocolate chips (reserve a few chips for the top). Spoon the batter into the baking dish and spread it to the edges. Top with the reserved chocolate chips.

4 Bake until the top is lightly golden, about 30 minutes. Remove from the oven and let cool for 10 to 15 minutes before serving.

5 Once cooled, store the baked oatmeal in a covered airtight container for two to three days or freeze for four to six weeks.

Whipped Cottage Cheese Parfait

+ SOY & PHYTOESTROGENS + PROTEIN + FIBER + CALCIUM

Makes 4 servings

When I first heard of whipped cottage cheese, I was skeptical. Cottage cheese is convenient and delicious on its own, so would taking the time to whip it in a food processor be worth it? The answer is a resounding yes! Creamy and smooth, whipped cottage cheese adds a layer of pleasure and satisfaction to this breakfast parfait, making it well worth the effort. It's also a great option for anyone who has previously shied away from cottage cheese because of its lumpy texture.

---

2 cups (420 g) 2% cottage cheese (see note)

1 cup (240 ml) Very Berry Chia Jam (page 125)

1 cup (115 g) fresh or thawed frozen raspberries, blackberries, or blueberries

⅓ cup (30 g) sweetened or unsweetened toasted coconut

---

1 Place the cottage cheese in a blender or food processor and mix until smooth, scraping down the sides of the blender as needed.

2 In a parfait glass or other wide-mouth jar, layer the cottage cheese, chia jam, and berries. Repeat the layers two more times. Make three more parfaits with the remaining ingredients.

3 Sprinkle the toasted coconut on top and enjoy!

4 The parfaits will keep in the refrigerator, covered, for 24 hours.

In a hurry? Swap Greek yogurt or quark for the cottage cheese. Quark is a favorite in some European countries including Germany; it's technically a cheese but closer in taste and texture to yogurt.

Note: If you're watching your salt intake, look for reduced-sodium cottage cheese.

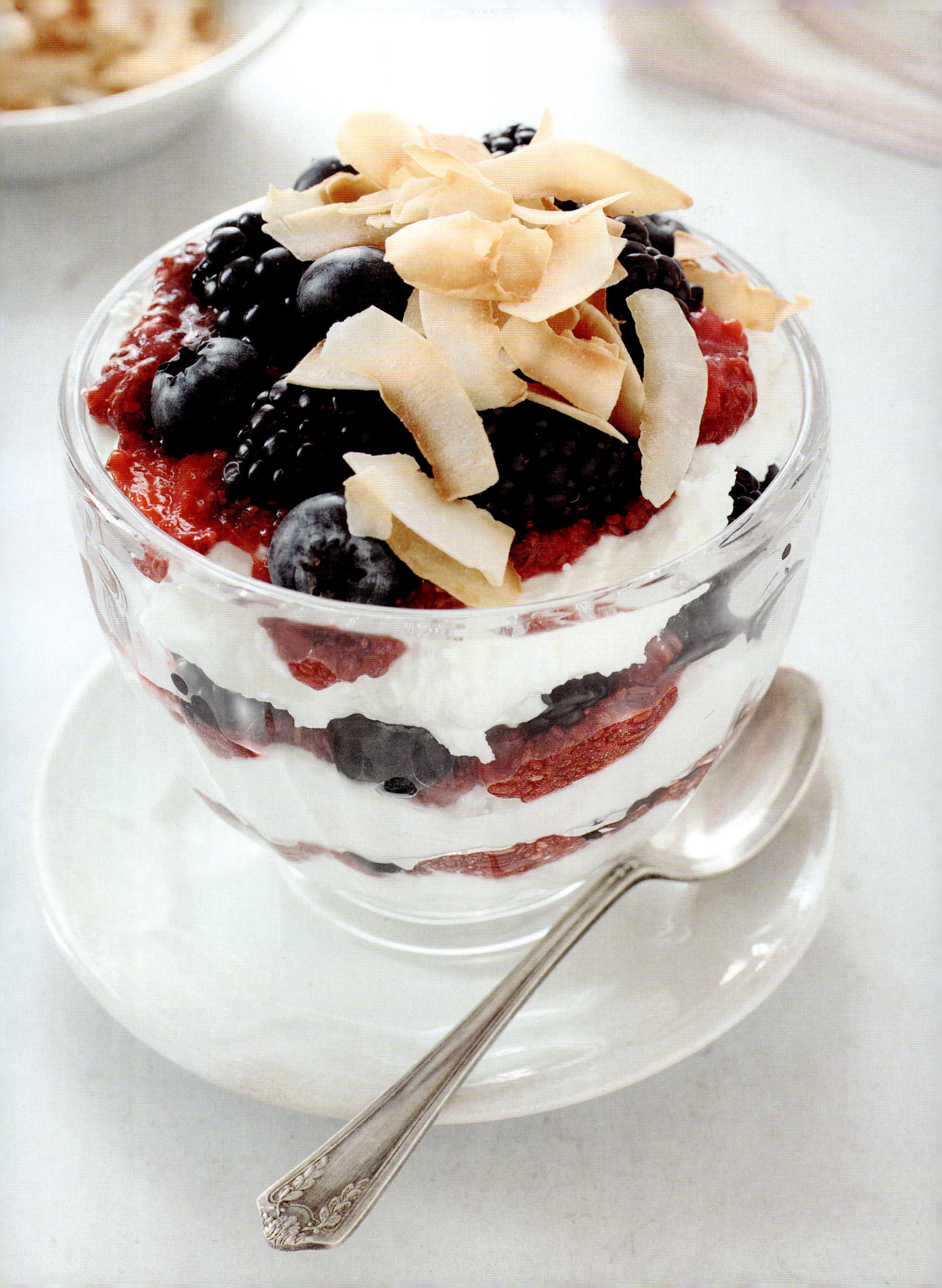

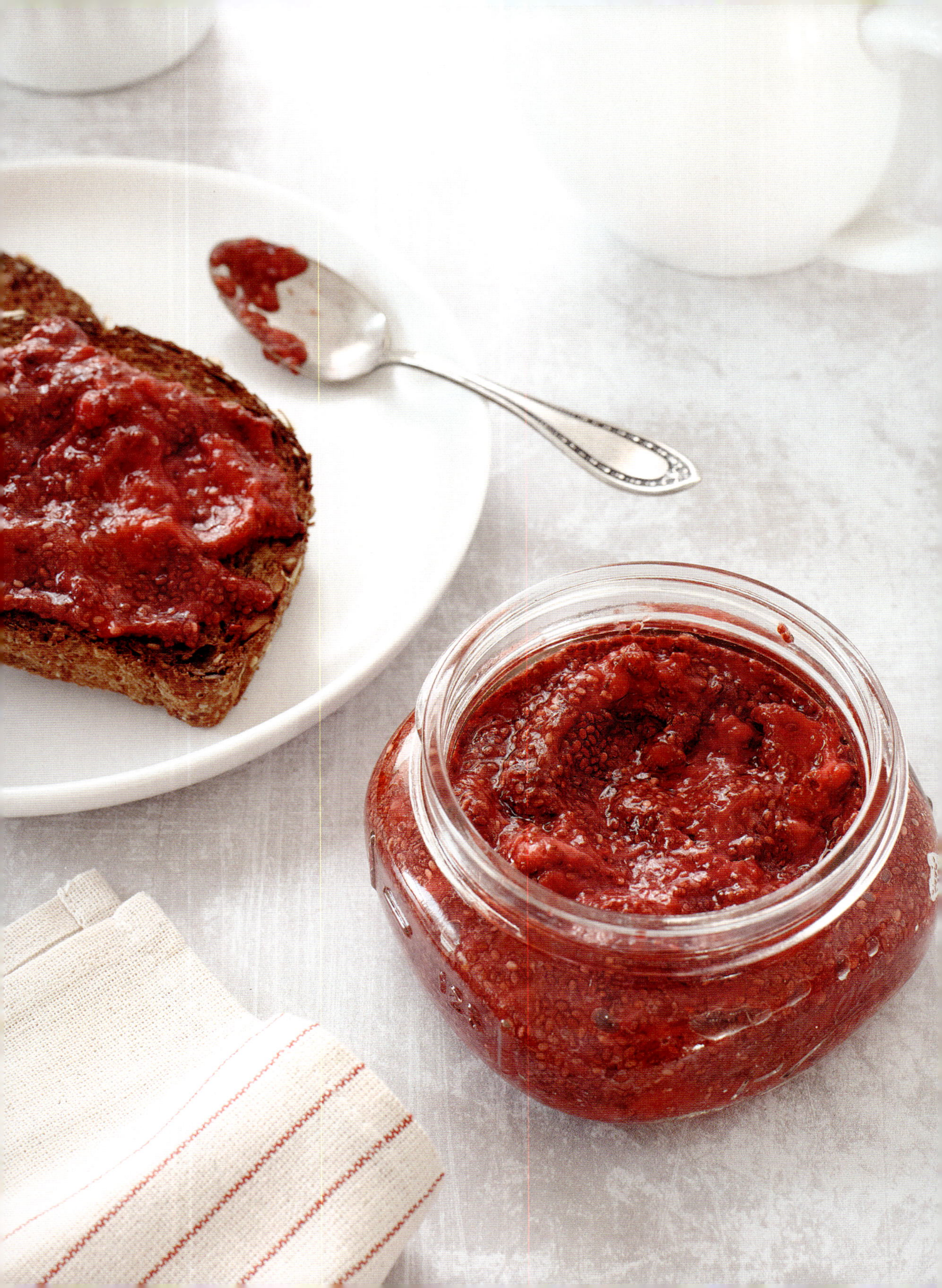

Very Berry Chia Jam

+ FIBER + CALCIUM + OMEGA-3

Makes 2 cups (500 ml)

I love finding new ways to add a burst of berry flavor to my go-to breakfast foods. This chia seed berry jam cooks up quickly and adds fiber, calcium, and satisfaction to oatmeal, PB&J, yogurt, or cottage cheese. As the "jam" cooks and then cools, the seeds will swell and act like pectin, the gel-like substance used in jams and preserves. Chia seeds may be a relatively new addition to our modern grocery store shelves, but they have a rich history. Native to Mexico and parts of South America, these small seeds were once used as currency during the Aztec empire. You'll find chia seeds in white and black varieties, but nutritionally they're very similar. Chia seeds have an impressive fiber content, making up 33 percent of the seeds' nutritional value. Like flax, chia seeds are an excellent source of ALA, the plant-based parent to the health-promoting omega-3 fatty acids. But unlike flax, chia seeds don't need to be ground to access these health-promoting fats.

2½ cups (350 g) frozen strawberries or any red berries

¼ cup (60 ml) water

1 teaspoon pure vanilla extract

1 tablespoon maple syrup or honey

¼ cup (40 g) chia seeds

1 Combine the berries, water, vanilla, and maple syrup in a medium saucepan and cook over low heat until the berries are soft, about 5 minutes. Using a fork, mash until no whole berries remain.

2 Stir in the chia seeds and continue to simmer, uncovered on low, until the chia seeds start to swell, 3 to 5 minutes.

3 Remove from the heat and pour the mixture into a mason jar or heatproof glass dish to cool.

4 Once cooled, enjoy the jam on top of oatmeal or toast.

5 The jam can be refrigerated, covered in an airtight container, for up to five days.

Pumpkin Smoothie Bowl

+ **SOY & PHYTOESTROGENS** + **PROTEIN** + **FIBER** + **CALCIUM** + **OMEGA-3**

Makes 2 servings

Who needs a pumpkin spice latte when you can have a PSL-inspired meal that's nutritious and satisfying? Rich in fiber and potassium, pumpkin should be on your midlife menu all year round. The Greek yogurt and soy milk add protein, calcium, and creaminess to this satisfying meal, while the flax teams up with soy milk for a phytoestrogen one-two punch.

---

1 can (15 ounces/425 g) pumpkin puree (see note)

1 cup (235 g) plain Greek yogurt

1 medium banana, peeled

¼ cup (60 ml) soy milk

1 tablespoon honey or maple syrup

2 teaspoons pumpkin pie spice

1 teaspoon pure vanilla extract

¼ cup (30 g) pumpkin seeds

2 tablespoons ground flax

2 tablespoons chopped walnuts

---

1 Combine the pumpkin puree, yogurt, banana, soy milk, honey, pumpkin pie spice, and vanilla in a blender. Mix until smooth.

2 Divide the mixture evenly between two bowls and top with the pumpkin seeds, flax, and walnuts. Serve immediately.

Note: Canned pureed pumpkin is different from pumpkin pie filling, which is usually seasoned and sweetened. Be sure you use the former for this recipe.

In a hurry? Make this the night before and refrigerate for a quick and satisfying breakfast. Add the toppings just before serving.

Variation

SMOOTHIE: If you prefer a thinner texture—that is, a drinkable smoothie instead of a spoonable bowl—use 1 cup (240 ml) of soy milk and reduce the Greek yogurt to ¾ cup (175 g).

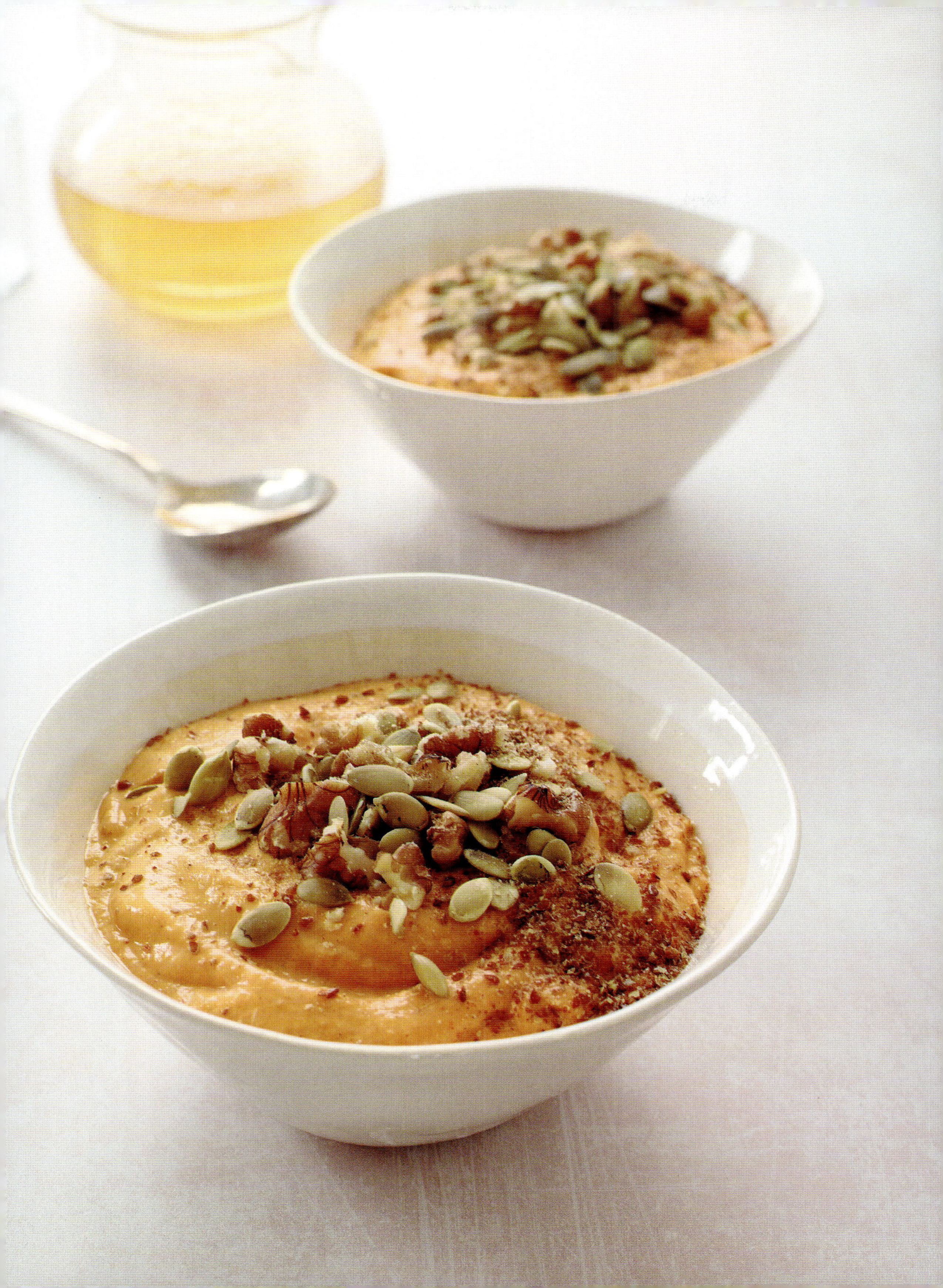

IS THERE A "BEST" MILK?

Most nondairy milk beverages are fortified with calcium and vitamin D, but only soy milk provides hot-flash-fighting phytoestrogens in the form of isoflavones. Unlike other plant-based milks, soy milk also provides 7 g of protein.

But the type of milk you use doesn't really matter that much because for most adults, milk is not a primary source of nutrition. In other words, you don't have to drink milk at all, but if you do, choose what you enjoy! Depending on your gentle nutrition goals in menopause, the type you choose might make a difference:

- Cow milk and soy milk are both sources of protein and can add to your daily protein goals.
- Soy milk is a source of phytoestrogens and unsaturated fats.
- Almond and oat milk may be easier to digest for people who are sensitive to dairy and soy.
- Almost all milks are fortified with calcium and vitamin D.

Menopause is hard enough; don't make it harder by overthinking what kind of milk or milk beverage is best!

Savory Sweet Potato Egg Bites

+ PROTEIN + FIBER

Makes 6 servings

One of the things I've come to appreciate is a savory breakfast like these sweet potato and egg bites. Sweet potatoes and spinach offer a heart-healthy dose of potassium while the feta adds a hint of creamy, salt-kissed satisfaction. Don't be fooled into thinking these egg bites are only for breakfast, though, because they make a perfect side dish to any meal. I often eat these with a salad or as a snack during the day.

Extra virgin olive oil, for greasing the muffin cups

2 medium sweet potatoes, peeled, cooked, and mashed

4 large eggs

½ teaspoon garlic powder

¼ teaspoon fine sea salt

1 small handful roughly chopped fresh spinach

¼ cup (40 g) crumbled feta cheese

---

1 Preheat the oven to 400°F (200°C). Lightly grease six muffin cups with the oil. You can also use muffin liners for easy cleanup.

2 Place the sweet potato in a medium bowl. In a small bowl, whisk together the eggs, garlic powder, salt, spinach, and feta. Add the egg mixture to the sweet potato and mix well to incorporate.

3 Divide the sweet potato–egg mixture evenly among the six prepared muffin cups, then bake until the tops are lightly golden brown, 20 to 22 minutes.

4 Remove from the oven and let cool for 5 minutes before serving.

5 Store leftovers in a covered dish in the refrigerator for up to three days. Reheat in a preheated oven (350°F/175°C) for 8 to 10 minutes.

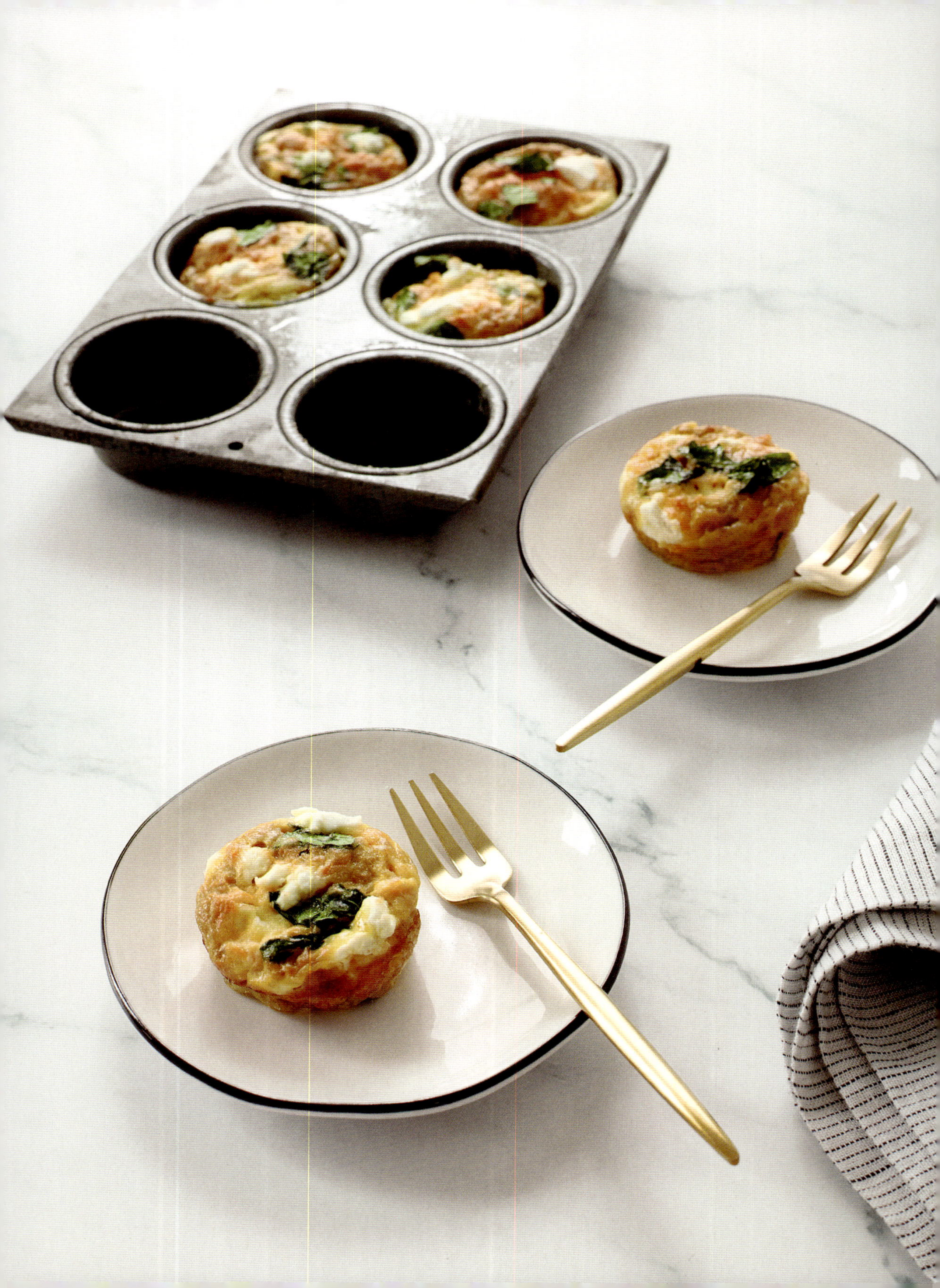

Undiet It! Sweet Potatoes versus White Potatoes

Do sweet potatoes have more sugar than white potatoes do? Not really. Compared side by side, there's little difference in carbohydrate and fiber content. White potatoes provide an impressive dose of potassium while sweet potatoes bring beta-carotene to the table. What about the glycemic index (GI), a measurement of how quickly a food raises blood sugar levels? Both white potatoes and sweet potatoes can have a GI that ranges from low to high, depending on how they're cooked. In other words, lead with satisfaction and don't worry about choosing the "best" potato.

Tofu Scramble

+ SOY & PHYTOESTROGENS + PROTEIN + FIBER + CALCIUM

Makes 4 servings

Scrambled eggs are easy to make, and this tofu scramble is no different. Enjoy it for breakfast, lunch, or dinner. The turmeric and nutritional yeast give the scramble a punch of color and added flavor that will make you think, "I can't believe these aren't eggs!" Texture is key here—be sure to press the tofu as directed to remove the excess liquid. For breakfast on the go, try adding a few spoonfuls of the scramble to a tortilla and top with salsa and cheese for a breakfast burrito.

---

1 package (14 ounces/397 g) extra-firm tofu, drained

1 small red onion, peeled

1 medium tomato, stemmed

1 small handful fresh spinach

⅓ cup (80 ml) soy milk

1 tablespoon nutritional yeast

1 teaspoon garlic powder

1 teaspoon ground turmeric

Pinch of chili powder (optional)

Fine sea salt and black pepper

1 tablespoon extra virgin olive oil

---

1 Remove the block of tofu from the packaging, wrap it in several layers of paper towel (or a tea towel), and place it on a plate. Place a heavy pan on top of it so that the tofu drains and expels water for at least 15 minutes (see page 135).

2 Meanwhile, dice the onion and tomato, then roughly chop the spinach. Set aside.

3 In a medium bowl, whisk together the soy milk, nutritional yeast, garlic powder, turmeric, and chili powder, if using. Season with a pinch of salt and black pepper.

continued

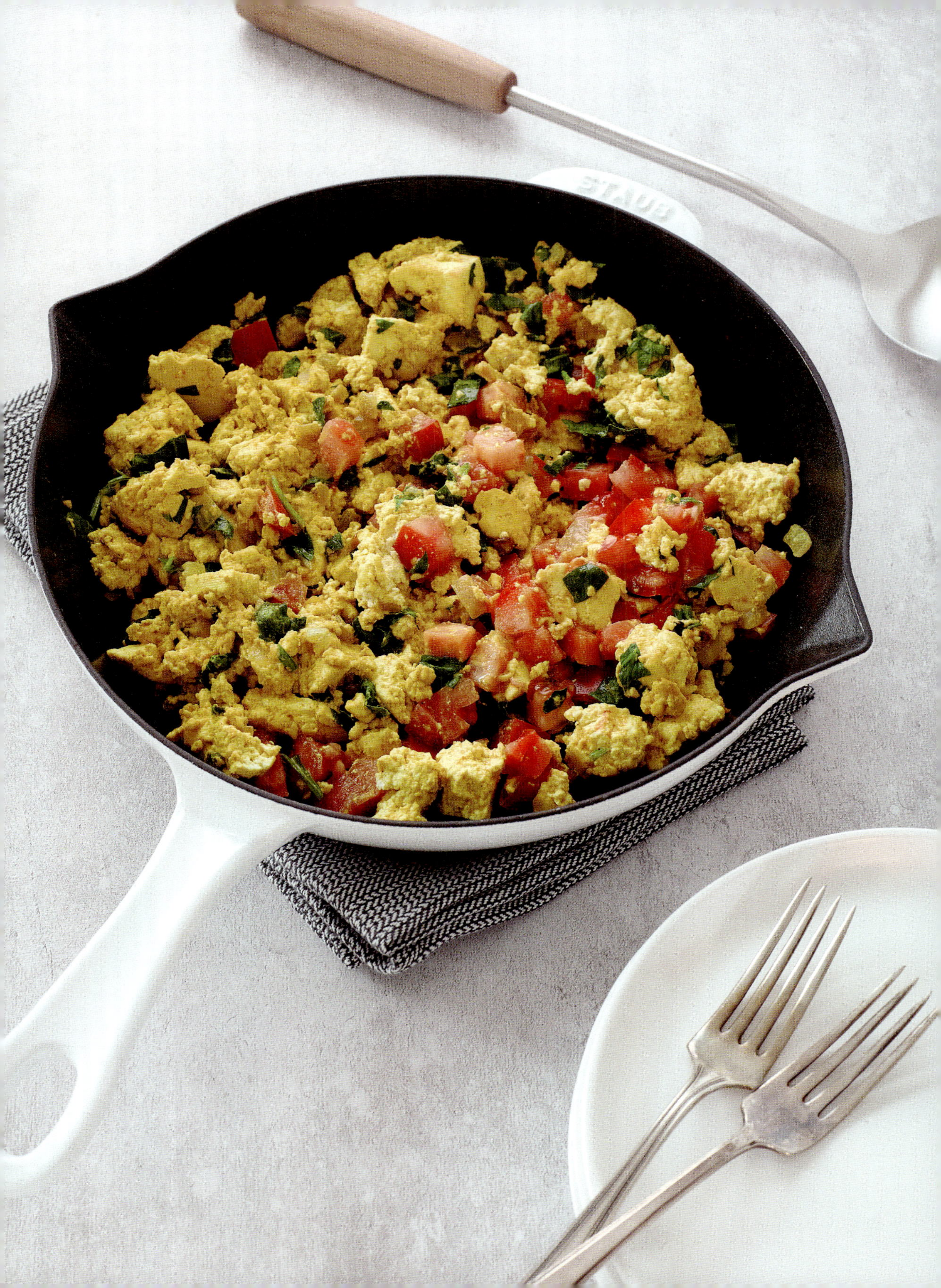
STAUB

4 When the tofu has almost finished draining, heat the oil in a medium skillet over medium heat. Add the onion and cook, stirring occasionally, until translucent, 3 to 4 minutes. Unwrap the tofu and loosely crumble it into the pan. Let it cook with the onion until the tofu is lightly golden, 2 to 3 minutes. Reduce the heat to low and stir in the soy milk mixture. Simmer, stirring frequently to prevent the tofu from sticking to the pan and burning, until it resembles the texture of scrambled eggs, 4 to 5 minutes.

5 Add the diced tomato and spinach and stir until the spinach is just wilted, 3 to 4 minutes. Serve immediately or let cool and store in the refrigerator, covered in an airtight container, for two to three days. Reheat on the stovetop for 3 to 5 minutes.

In a hurry? Prepare the cooked tofu through step 3, let cool, and store it overnight in the refrigerator. In the morning, reheat it and add the spinach and tomato as directed.

TYPES OF TOFU

All tofu is made from soybeans, but not all tofu is created equal. Most recipes that use tofu will specify the type required, but here's a quick description of the most common types and how they're used.

Silken Tofu

- **Texture:** Soft, creamy, and custard-like.
- **Flavor:** Mild and subtly sweet, although you'll sometimes find fruit-flavored varieties of this tofu, especially in Asian grocery stores.
- **Use:** Ideal for smoothies, desserts, dressings, and sauces. It blends smoothly, making it perfect for creamy and blended dishes.
- **Cooking:** No cooking needed; used directly from the package.

Soft Tofu

- **Texture:** Slightly firmer than silken but still delicate.
- **Flavor:** Mild with a slightly more pronounced bean taste than silken.
- **Use:** Best for soups (like miso soup) or in dips.
- **Cooking:** Handle gently to maintain its shape. It can be lightly pan-fried or simmered in soups.

Firm Tofu

- **Texture:** Holds its shape well, slightly dense.
- **Flavor:** Mild and bean-like.
- **Use:** Extremely versatile—great for stir-frying, baking, grilling, and scrambling.
- **Cooking:** Press out excess water (see Cooking Tips) for a firmer texture. It can be marinated, baked, or fried.

Extra-Firm Tofu

- **Texture:** Very dense and meaty.
- **Flavor:** More concentrated soybean taste.
- **Use:** Ideal for dishes needing a hearty texture, like kebabs, or when you want it to hold up well to vigorous cooking.
- **Cooking:** Press to remove excess moisture. Like firm tofu, it can be marinated, grilled, baked, or stir-fried.

Cooking Tips

- **Pressing tofu:** For firmer varieties, wrap the tofu block in several layers of paper towels and place it on a plate. Place a heavy pan on top to press out excess water for at least 15 minutes. This simple process yields a better texture and more flavor absorption. Alternatively, freezing tofu before unwrapping can expedite this process.
- **Marinating:** Tofu is like a sponge—it loves to soak up flavors. Marinate it for a minimum of 15 minutes before cooking.
- **Storing:** To store uncooked tofu, keep it in water in the refrigerator and change the water daily to keep it fresh.

Nourishing Soups and Stews

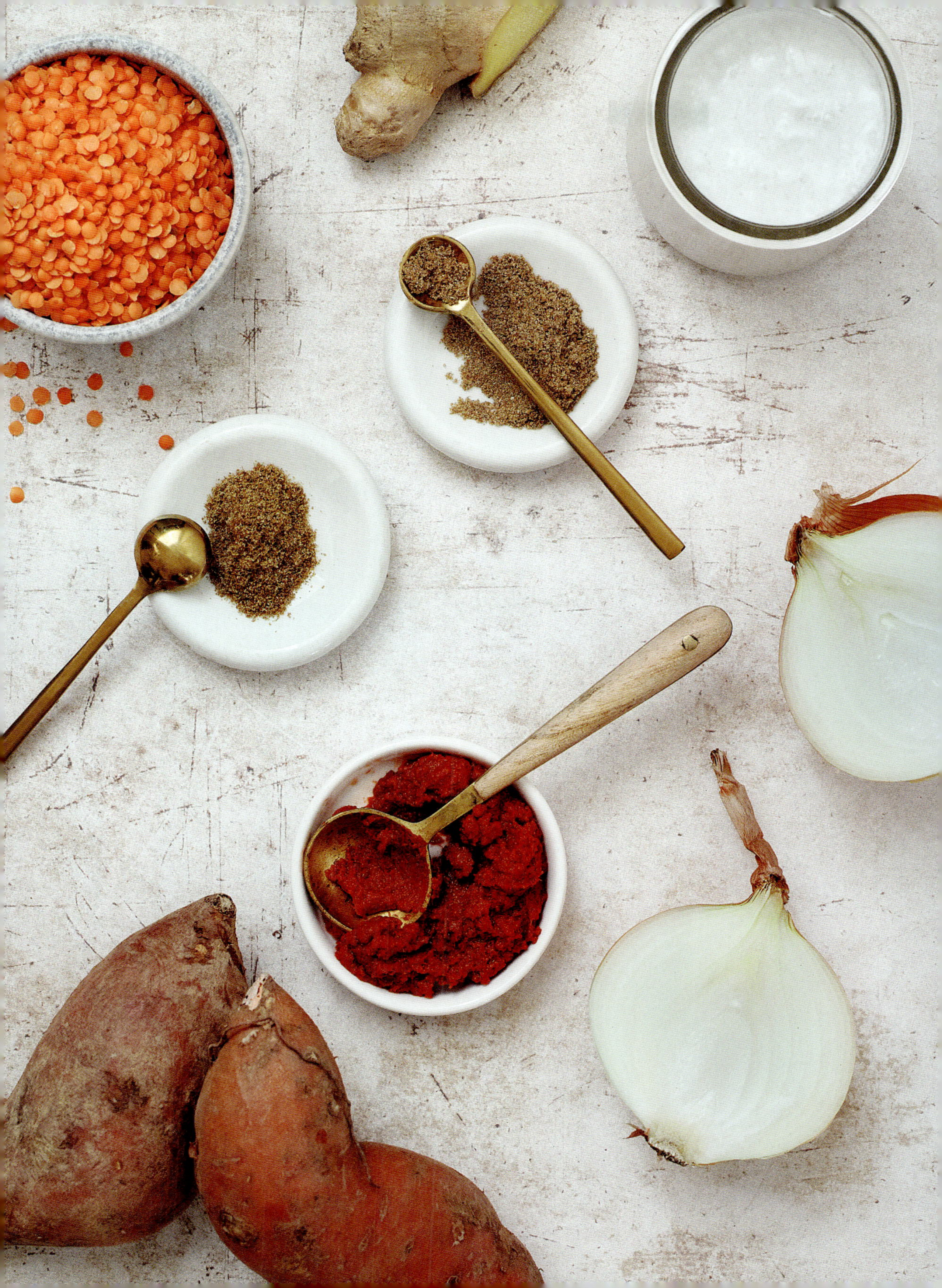

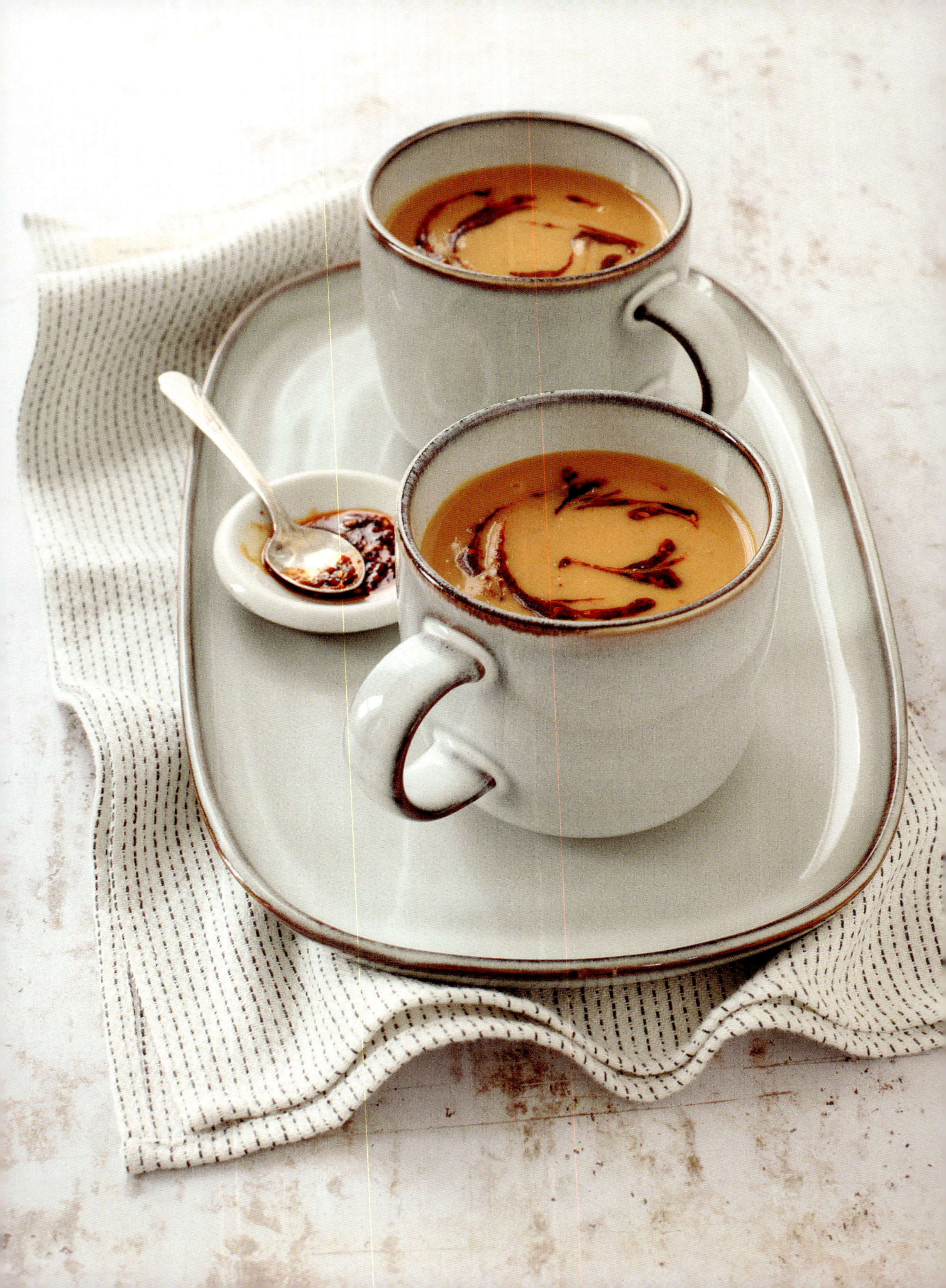

Thai Lentil and Sweet Potato Soup

+ PROTEIN + FIBER

Makes 4 servings

This comforting soup is easy to make, perfect for busy weeknights or lazy weekends. Lentils and sweet potatoes provide protein and fiber, while red curry paste, ginger, and cumin balance the sweetness of the potatoes and the creaminess of coconut milk. Serve with warm bread for added satisfaction.

---

2 teaspoons coconut oil
1 medium onion, diced
2 teaspoons grated fresh ginger
1 teaspoon ground coriander
½ teaspoon ground cumin
1 to 2 tablespoons red curry paste
4 cups (950 ml) chicken or vegetable broth
2 large sweet potatoes, diced
1 cup (190 g) red lentils, rinsed and drained
½ teaspoon fine sea salt
¾ cup (180 ml) light coconut milk
Chili crisp, for garnish

---

1 Warm the coconut oil in a large pot over medium heat. Add the onion, stir, and cook until translucent, 3 to 4 minutes. Add the ginger, coriander, and cumin and let them warm, stirring until fragrant, 1 to 2 minutes.

2 Add the red curry paste and continue to stir for another minute before adding the broth, sweet potatoes, lentils, and salt. Bring to a boil, then reduce the heat to low and simmer until the sweet potatoes are tender and the lentils are soft, 20 to 25 minutes.

3 Stir in the coconut milk and continue simmering on low until creamy and well combined, 2 to 3 minutes. Remove from the heat. Using an immersion blender, puree the soup until smooth.

4 Ladle into bowls and serve immediately. For extra heat, top with chili crisp.

5 You can store leftover soup in an airtight container and refrigerate for four to five days. For longer storage, freeze the soup in individual portions using freezer-safe containers. The soup can be frozen for up to three months.

Pea Soup
with Feta and Mint

+ FIBER + CALCIUM

Makes 4 servings

Hold the hot flashes! Although delicious as a warm dish, this soup can also be enjoyed cold, making it a welcome meal on days when the temperature outside (or inside) is heating up. Not to be confused with split pea soup, which uses dried peas, whole green peas are the star of this recipe. Brightened up with fresh mint and salty feta cheese, this soup will quickly become your go-to meal when the temperatures soar.

---

2 tablespoons extra virgin olive oil

4 ribs celery, diced

2 cloves garlic, minced

1 medium onion, diced

4 cups (950 ml) chicken or vegetable broth

2 cups (290 g) fresh or frozen (unthawed) green peas

½ cup (75 g) crumbled feta cheese

¼ cup (15 g) chopped fresh mint

---

1 Warm the oil in a large pot over medium heat. Add the celery, garlic, and onion. Stirring occasionally, cook until the onion is soft and translucent, 3 to 5 minutes.

2 Add the broth and peas and bring to a boil, then reduce the heat to low and simmer, stirring occasionally, until the peas are soft, about 15 minutes.

3 Remove the soup from the heat and puree with an immersion blender until smooth. Top with the feta and mint before serving.

4 To enjoy this soup cold, allow it to cool to room temperature or refrigerate for 2 to 3 hours in an airtight container. Ladle the cold soup into serving bowls and garnish with the feta and mint before serving.

5 Store leftover soup in an airtight container in the refrigerator for four to five days. To reheat, warm it on the stove over medium-low heat, stirring occasionally, until heated through.

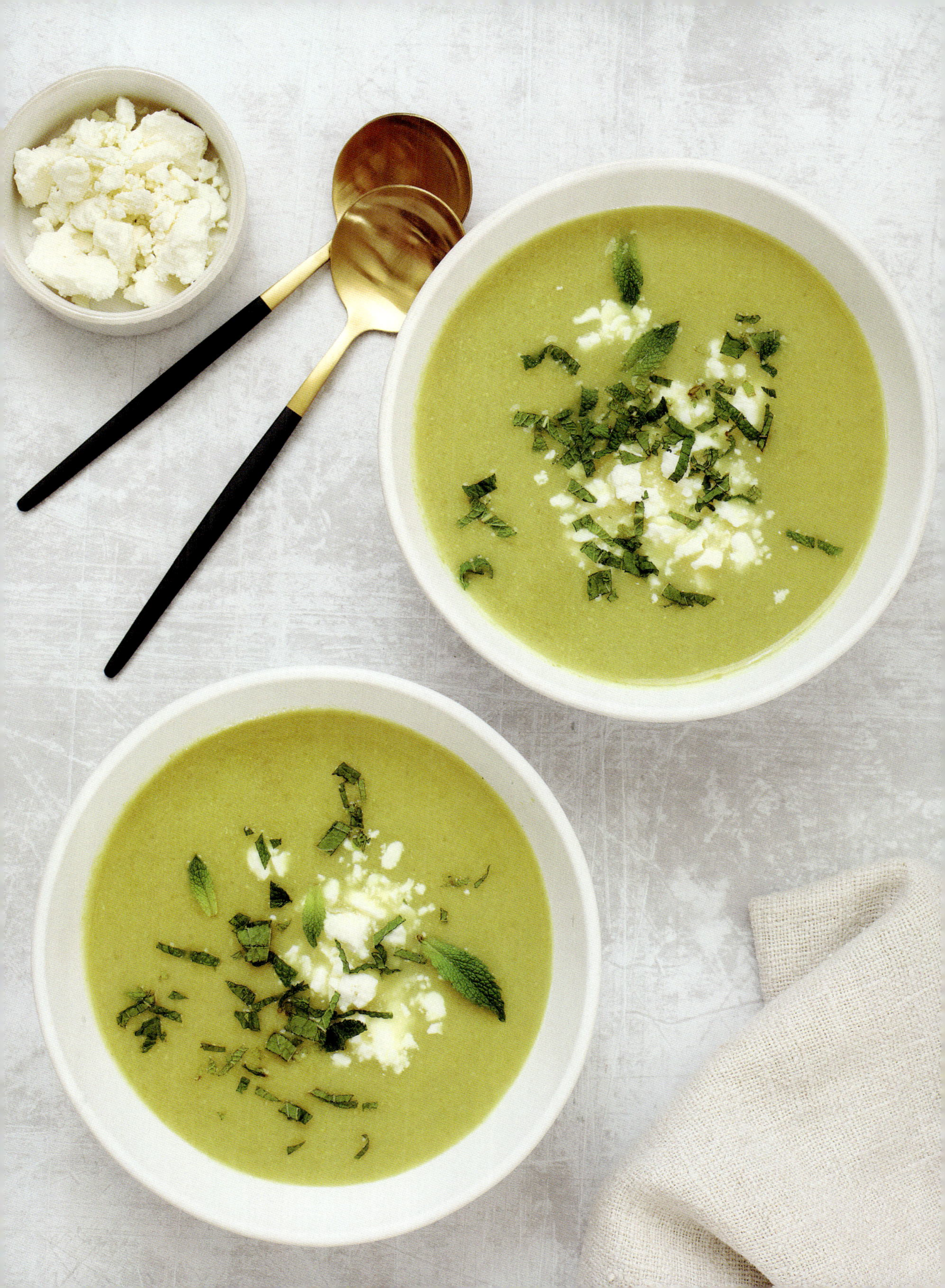

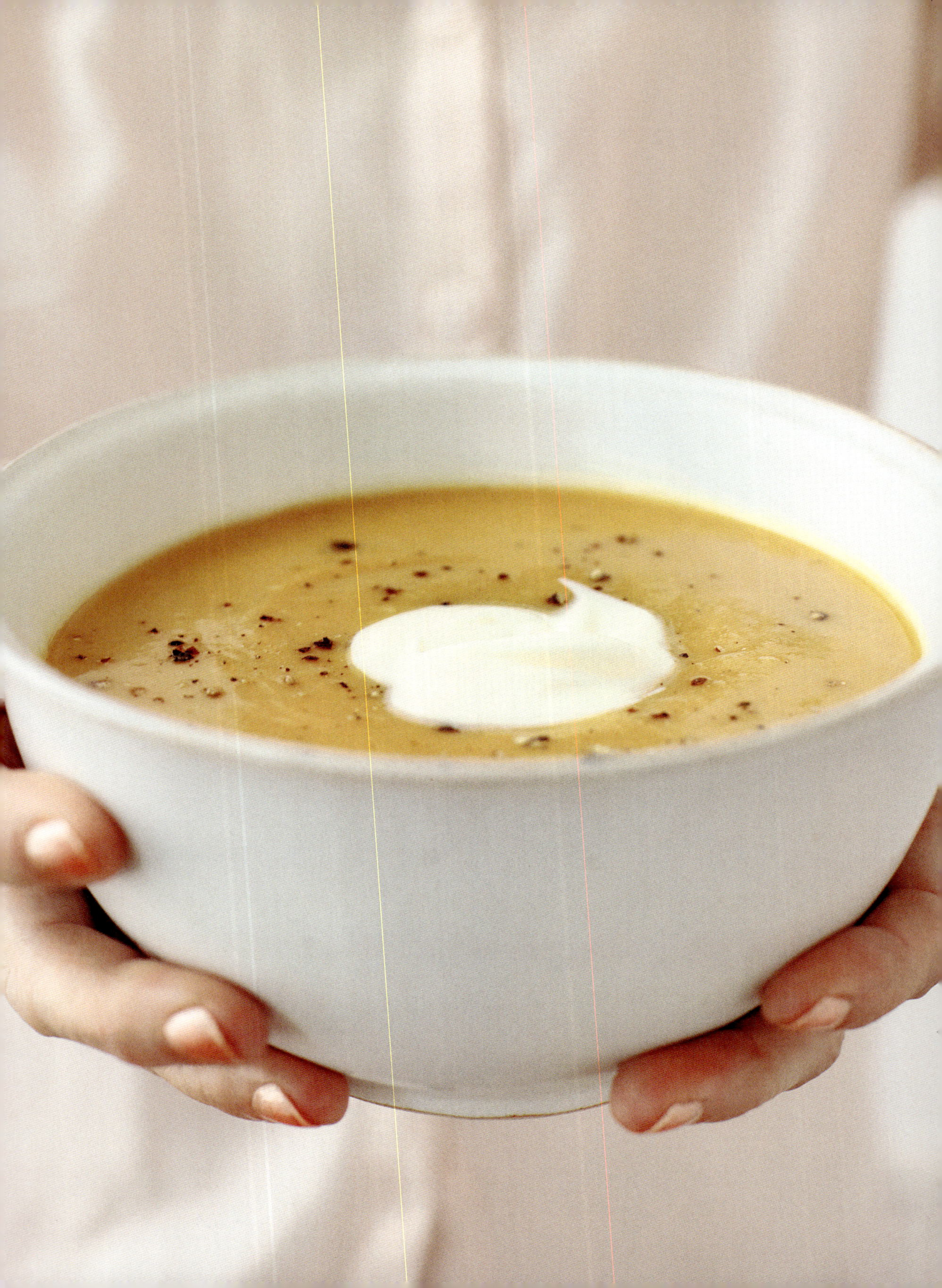

Ginger Squash and Red Lentil Soup

+ PROTEIN + FIBER

Makes 4 servings

Have you ever made something that was so easy and delicious that you found yourself wondering how you'd never made it before? That's the reaction I get all the time to this incredibly quick and easy soup. The lentils up the satisfaction factor by providing protein and fiber while the cumin and coriander give depth to this otherwise simple soup. If you love ginger as much as I do, feel free to grate some fresh ginger into the soup just before serving. For extra tang and creaminess, crumble feta cheese over the top or add a spoonful of crème fraîche.

- 1 tablespoon extra virgin olive oil
- 1 medium onion, diced
- 1 piece (2 inches/5 cm) fresh ginger, minced
- 2 teaspoons ground cumin
- 1 teaspoon ground coriander
- 1 medium butternut squash, peeled and cut into 1-inch (2.5 cm) cubes
- 1 cup (190 g) red lentils, rinsed and drained
- 5 cups (1.1 L) chicken or vegetable broth
- 1 teaspoon fine sea salt
- ½ teaspoon black pepper

---

1 Warm the oil in a large pot over medium heat. Add the onion and ginger, stirring occasionally, and cook until the onion is translucent and fragrant, 2 to 3 minutes. Stir in the cumin and coriander, cooking until the spices are fragrant, about 1 minute.

2 Mix in the squash and lentils, stirring to ensure they're well coated with the spices. Pour in the broth and bring the mixture to a boil, then reduce the heat to medium-low to maintain a simmer. Season with the salt and black pepper. Cover and cook until the lentils and squash are tender, about 30 minutes.

3 Divide the soup among four bowls and serve hot.

4 Store leftover soup in an airtight container in the refrigerator for four to five days. To reheat, warm it on the stove over medium-low heat, stirring occasionally, until heated through. It's common for soups made with red lentils to thicken after refrigeration. Add a splash of broth or water to adjust the consistency.

Tortilla Soup

+ PROTEIN + FIBER

Makes 6 servings

Whether you're feeding a small crowd or just a few people, the familiar Mexican-inspired flavors of this soup make it a reliable crowd-pleaser. The toppings are the best part, allowing everyone to adjust this soup to their own tastes. For an easy dinner, add the ingredients to your slow cooker in the morning and come home to a comforting meal that is almost ready to serve.

---

1 tablespoon extra virgin olive oil

1 medium onion, diced

2 cloves garlic, diced

1 red bell pepper, stemmed, seeded, and diced

4 cups (950 ml) chicken or vegetable broth

3 boneless, skinless chicken breasts

1 can (14½ ounces/411 g) diced tomatoes, with juices

1 can (15 ounces/425 g) black beans, rinsed and drained

1 can (15 ounces/425 g) kidney beans, rinsed and drained

1 cup (165 g) canned or frozen corn kernels

1½ tablespoons taco seasoning (1 packet)

½ teaspoon smoked paprika

½ teaspoon fine sea salt

¼ teaspoon black pepper

Tortilla chips, shredded cheese, pickled or fresh jalapeño slices, sour cream, avocado, and/or lime wedges, for serving

---

1 Warm the oil in a large pot over medium heat. Add the onion, garlic, and bell pepper and cook, stirring until the onion and bell pepper are softened, 3 to 4 minutes.

2 Add the broth, chicken, tomatoes, black beans, kidney beans, corn, taco seasoning, paprika, salt, and black pepper. Bring the soup to a boil, then reduce the heat to low and simmer for 20 to 25 minutes, until the flavors meld together and the chicken has reached an internal temperature of 165°F (74°C).

continued

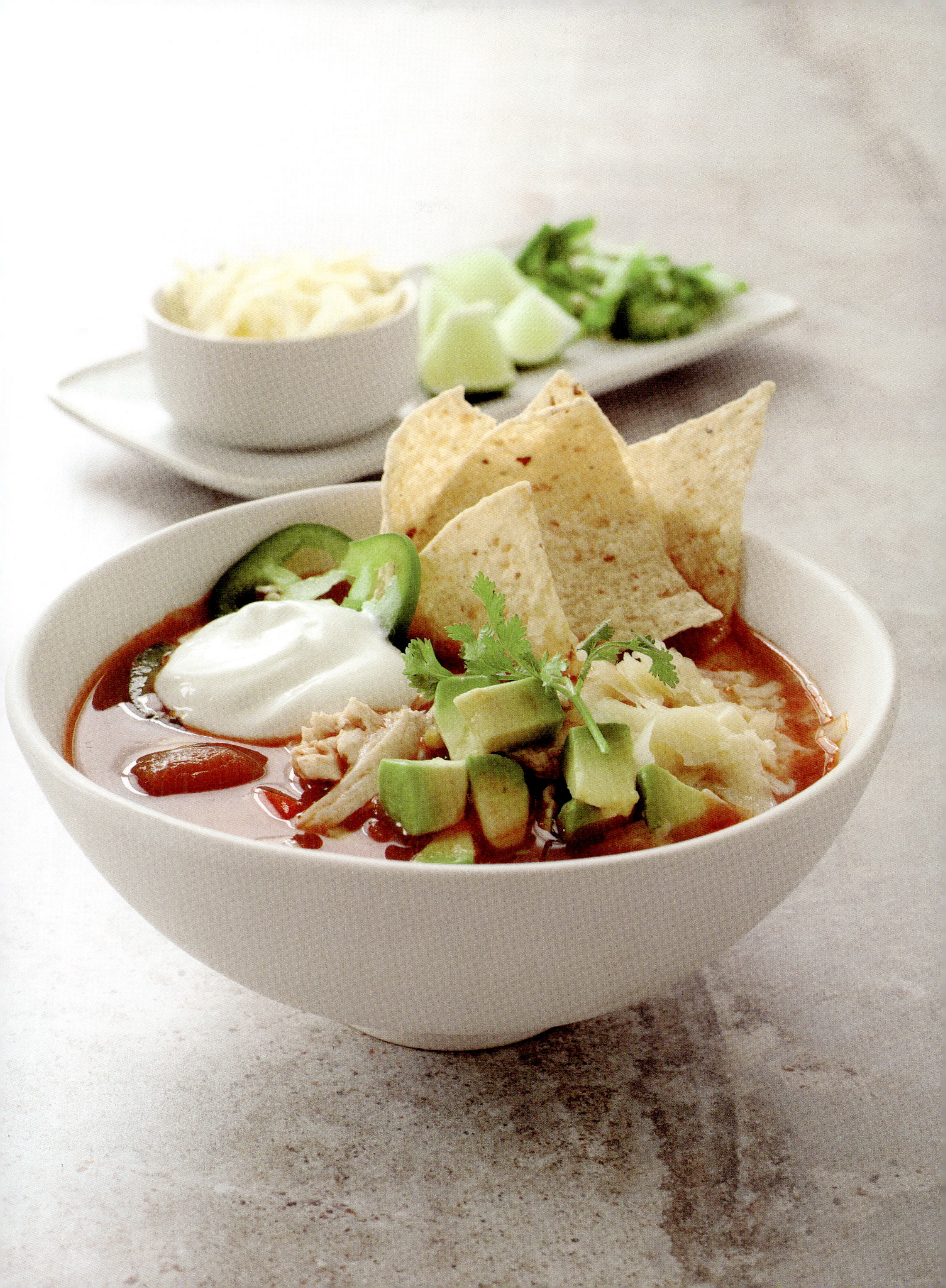

3 Carefully remove the chicken breasts from the soup and place them on a work surface or dinner plate. Using two forks, shred the chicken. Return the shredded chicken to the soup and simmer on low until warmed through, about 5 minutes.

4 Remove the soup from the heat and divide it among six bowls. Serve with the assorted toppings at the table so each person can customize their own bowl.

5 To freeze, portion soup (without toppings) into freezer-safe containers and freeze for up to three months. To reheat, thaw overnight in the refrigerator and heat on the stove or in the microwave until warmed through.

Variation

SLOW COOKER TORTILLA SOUP: If your slow cooker has a sauté function, follow the recipe as directed, cooking the soup on low for 6 to 8 hours or high for 3 to 4 hours. Otherwise, sauté the onion, garlic, and bell pepper in a skillet, then transfer to the slow cooker and continue with the recipe as directed, cooking for 6 to 8 hours on low or 3 to 4 hours on high.

Mushroom Lentil Stew

+ PROTEIN + FIBER + CALCIUM

Makes 2 servings

Mushroom fans will love this quick lentil stew that allows the earthy and comforting flavor of mushrooms to take center stage. Mushrooms are a source of beta-glucan, the special type of soluble fiber that's also found in oats and barley. Unlike other types of lentils, French green lentils retain their shape while soaking up the flavors of the broth. Serve this over mashed potatoes or rice for a more substantial meal.

---

1 tablespoon extra virgin olive oil

1 small onion, diced

2 cups (190 g) whole white mushrooms, trimmed and sliced (see note)

1 tablespoon low-sodium tamari or light soy sauce

⅔ cup (130 g) French green lentils, rinsed and drained

2 cups (475 ml) vegetable or chicken broth, plus more as needed

2 tablespoons chopped fresh thyme, or 2 teaspoons dried thyme

1 bunch Swiss chard, stemmed and roughly chopped

Fine sea salt and black pepper

Cooked rice or mashed potatoes, for serving

---

1 Warm the oil in a large pan over medium heat. Add the onion, stir, and cook until translucent, 2 to 3 minutes. Add the mushrooms and tamari and cook, stirring constantly, until the mushrooms start to soften, 2 to 3 minutes. Add the lentils, broth, and the thyme. Bring to a boil, then reduce heat to low and let simmer, covered, for 20 minutes. Remove the lid and test the lentils. They should be soft and mostly cooked. If not, add another ¼ cup (60 ml) of broth and cook for another 5 minutes.

continued

2 Once the lentils are soft and most of the broth (but not all) has reduced, add the Swiss chard and 1 to 2 tablespoons of broth, just enough to make a thin, gravy-like sauce. Stir, cover, and let simmer for a few minutes until the chard has softened. Season with salt and pepper to taste.

3 Serve the stew over rice or mashed potatoes, if desired.

Note: You can use any variety of mushrooms in this stew or a mix of your favorites. Note that the amount of broth needed will vary slightly depending on the water content of the mushrooms.

Feast on This!

Did you know that mushrooms are one of the few foods that can provide us with vitamin D? Mushrooms grown outside and exposed to sunlight or those grown under UV lights can be a good source of dietary vitamin D. Amounts vary by type of mushroom, but many can provide more than 400 IU of vitamin D per 100 g.

EXPLORING THE WORLD OF LENTILS

Lentils are a powerhouse of nutrition. Rich in the key ingredients of protein and fiber, lentils are also a good source of iron, which can help keep your energy up. I love the versatility of lentils, especially in soups and stews. They absorb flavors beautifully and can be pureed or used whole, making them perfect for a wide range of dishes. Here's a guide to understanding the different types of lentils and how to incorporate them into your meals.

- **Brown lentils:** The most common variety, brown lentils have an earthy flavor. They hold their shape well but can become mushy if overcooked. Perfect for soups and stews, they typically cook in 20 to 30 minutes.
- **Green lentils:** Slightly peppery in taste, green lentils retain their firm texture even after cooking. They are ideal for salads and side dishes. Like brown lentils, they cook in 20 to 30 minutes.
- **Red and yellow lentils:** These lentils have a sweet, nutty flavor and are more commonly found in Middle Eastern and Indian dishes. They cook quickly (15 to 20 minutes) and tend to break down, making them perfect for dahls and purees and for thickening soups.
- **Black (Beluga) lentils:** Named for their resemblance to caviar, these lentils have a rich, earthy flavor. They are great for adding texture to salads and side dishes. Cook them for 25 to 30 minutes, until tender but not mushy.
- **French green lentils:** Known for their slightly mineral-like, peppery flavor, these lentils hold their shape excellently. They cook in 25 to 30 minutes and are ideal in dishes where you want a firmer texture, such as the Lentil Salad with Roasted Carrots and Mushrooms (page 156).

Cooking Instructions

1. **Rinse and sort:** Always start by rinsing lentils under cold water. Sort through them to remove any small stones or debris. Drain well.
2. **Cook:** Combine 1 cup (190 g) lentils with 2 to 3 cups (475 to 700 ml) water in a large pot. Bring to a boil before reducing the heat and simmering uncovered for 20 to 25 minutes.
3. **Season:** Lentils absorb flavors well, so consider adding fresh or dried herbs, garlic, or onions to the cooking liquid. Salt or acidic ingredients can toughen the lentils, so don't add them until the lentils are fully cooked.
4. **Drain:** If there's excess water when the lentils are cooked, simply drain it off.

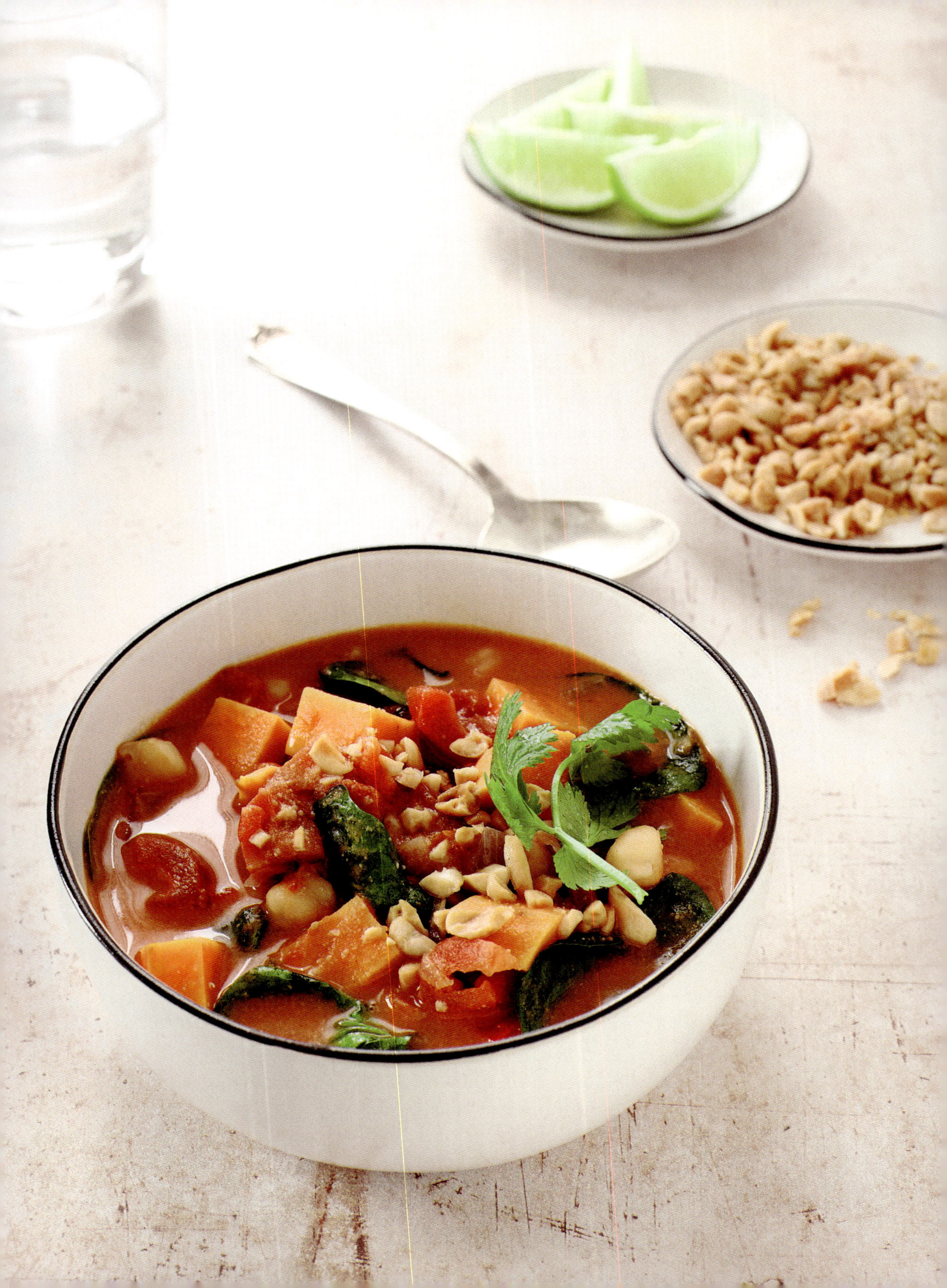

Savory Sweet Potato, Chickpea, and Peanut Stew

+ PROTEIN + FIBER

Makes 4 to 6 servings

Sweet, smoky, rich, and creamy—this stew is a hit with everyone. It's the ultimate comfort meal that's both nourishing and satisfying. Serve over cooked rice for extra heartiness.

---

1 tablespoon extra virgin olive oil

1 medium onion, diced

4 cloves garlic, minced

1 red or orange bell pepper, diced

1 large sweet potato, peeled and diced

1 can (28 ounces/800 g) diced tomatoes with juices

3 cups (700 ml) vegetable or chicken broth

½ cup (145 g) natural peanut butter

1½ teaspoons chili powder (optional)

1 teaspoon smoked paprika

1 can (15½ ounces/439 g) chickpeas, rinsed and drained

1 cup (30 g) packed baby spinach

¾ cup (180 ml) coconut milk

Fine sea salt and black pepper

¼ cup (40 g) crushed roasted peanuts

Fresh cilantro, for garnish

1 lime, cut into wedges

---

1 Warm the oil in a large pot over medium heat. Add the onion, stir, and cook until translucent, 2 to 3 minutes. Add the garlic and bell pepper and cook, stirring occasionally, until soft and fragrant, 2 to 3 minutes.

2 Stir in the sweet potato, tomatoes with juices, broth, peanut butter, chili powder, if using, and paprika. Bring to a boil, then cover and reduce the heat to low, and simmer until the sweet potatoes are tender, about 20 minutes.

3 Add the chickpeas, spinach, and coconut milk. Stir and cook until the spinach has wilted and the chickpeas are heated through, 3 to 5 minutes. Season to taste with salt and black pepper.

4 Ladle the stew into bowls, garnish with the peanuts and cilantro, and serve with lime wedges on the side.

Midlife Mains

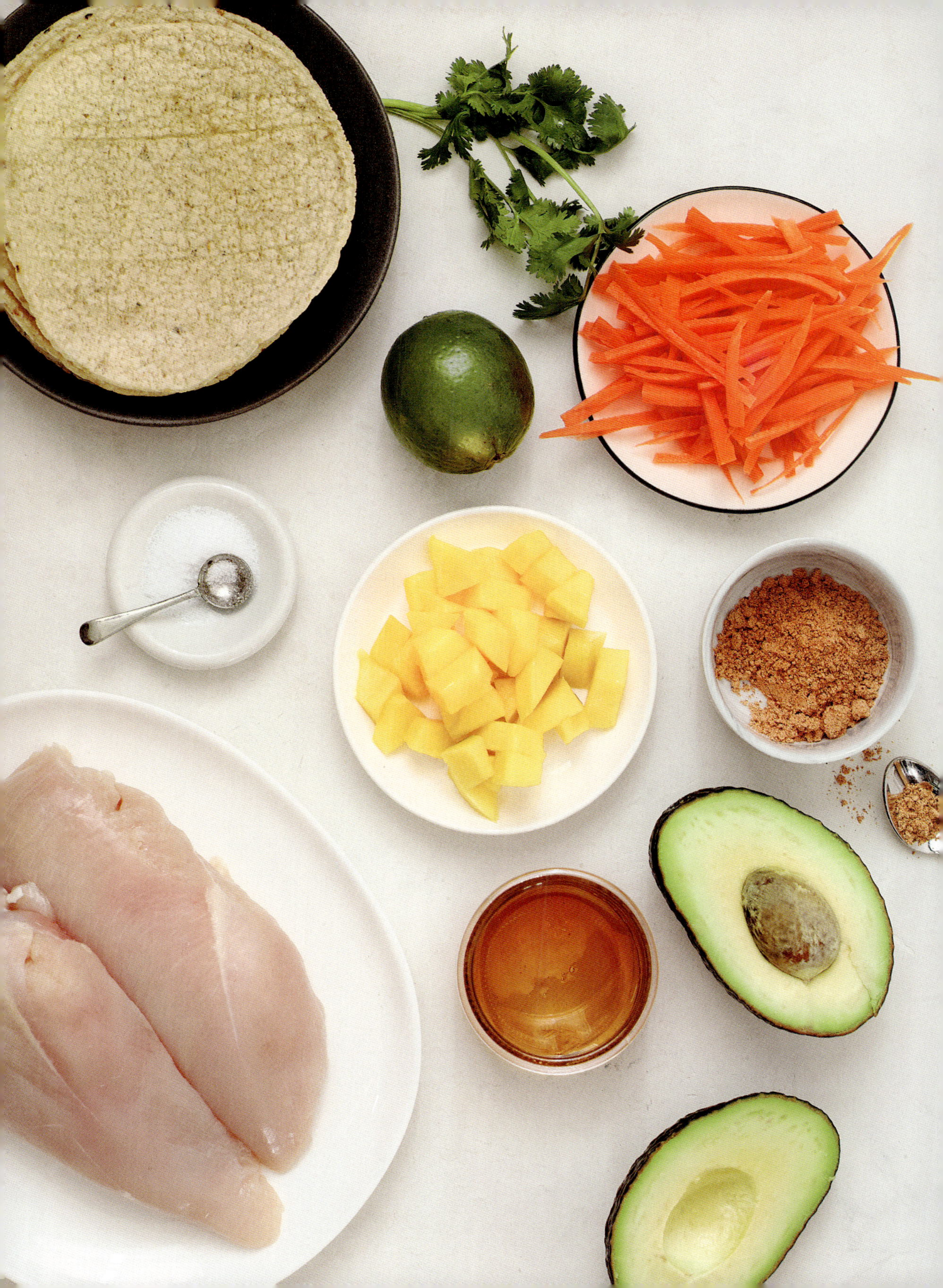

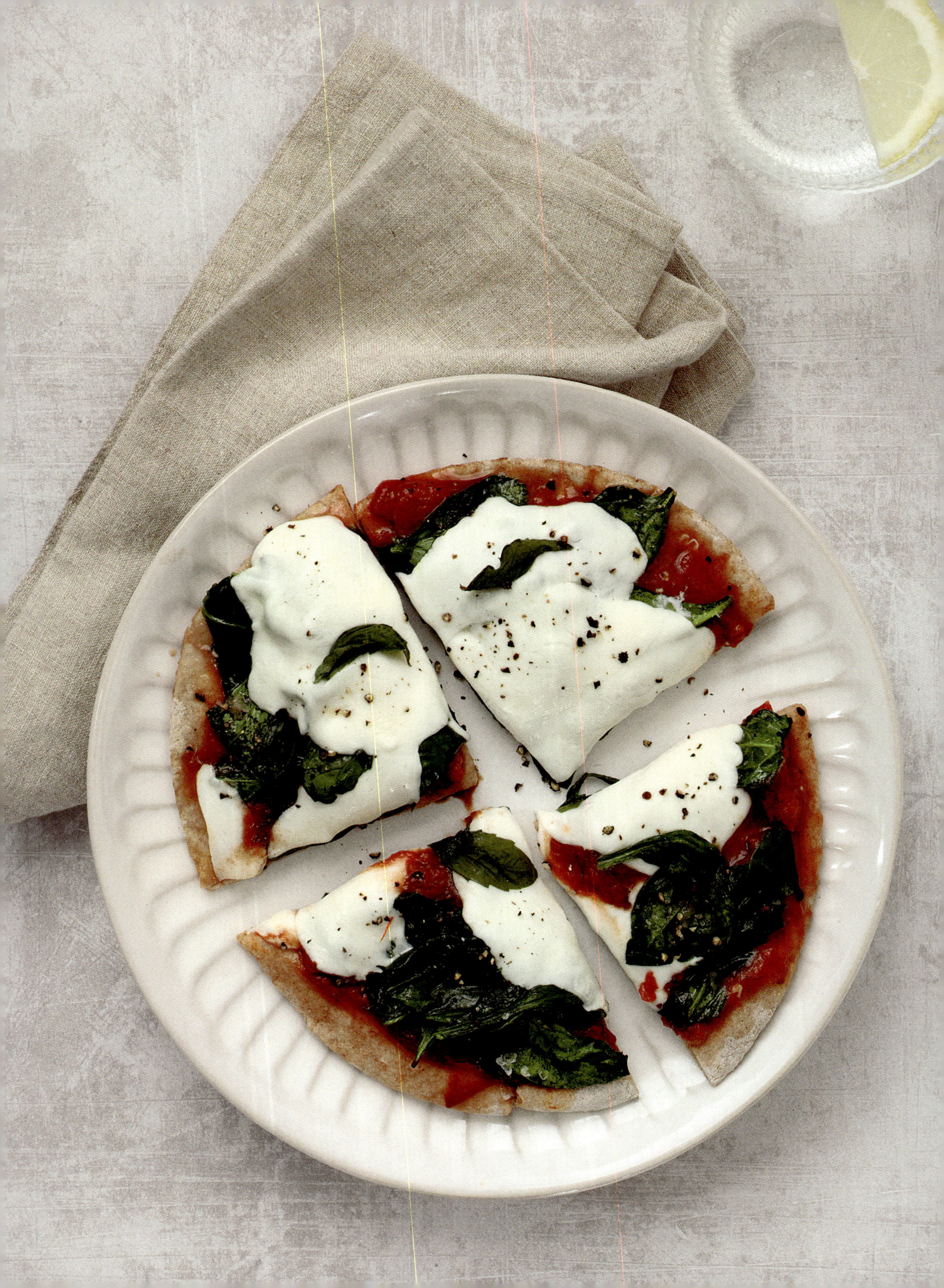

Spinach and Mozzarella Pita Pizza

+ PROTEIN + FIBER + CALCIUM

Makes 1 serving

One of the things I enjoy about working from home is making lunches for one—that I don't have to share with anyone. I used to treat lunch as an afterthought, but as an intuitive eater, I now really welcome the opportunity for a moment of pleasure and satisfaction in the middle of my day. This spinach and mozzarella pizza is a lunch I always enjoy, and the added benefit is that it's rich in calcium from both the spinach and the mozzarella.

½ teaspoon extra virgin olive oil

2 cups (60g) fresh spinach, roughly chopped

Fine sea salt and black pepper

¼ cup (60 ml) marinara or tomato-based pasta sauce (for homemade, see page 158)

1 large pita

1 ounce (30 g) fresh mozzarella, sliced

Fresh basil leaves, for topping (optional)

---

1 Preheat the oven to 375°F (190°C).

2 Warm the oil in a medium skillet over medium heat. Add the spinach and cook, stirring occasionally, until just wilted, about 2 minutes. Remove from the heat and season with salt and black pepper.

3 Spread the marinara sauce evenly over the pita bread, leaving a small border around the edges. Place the cooked spinach, mozzarella, and basil, if using, and sprinkle some more pepper on top.

4 Place the pita pizza on a baking sheet and bake for 6 to 8 minutes, until the cheese is melted.

Lentil Salad
with Roasted Carrots and Mushrooms

+ PROTEIN + FIBER + CALCIUM

Makes 4 servings

The combination of earthy lentils, oyster mushrooms, sweet roasted carrots, and creamy goat cheese makes this a salad that truly eats like a meal. Along with the protein and fiber, the rich flavors of this warm lentil salad will hit the spot.

---

3 to 4 medium carrots, trimmed and sliced lengthwise

2 tablespoons extra virgin olive oil, plus more for drizzling

Fine sea salt and black pepper

1 cup (190 g) French lentils, rinsed and drained

4½ ounces (130 g) soft goat cheese

3 tablespoons plain Greek yogurt

2 tablespoons red wine vinegar

1 teaspoon Dijon mustard

5½ ounces (155 g) oyster mushrooms

3 tablespoons fresh flat-leaf parsley, chopped

---

1 Preheat the oven to 425°F (220°C).

2 In a medium bowl, toss the carrots with a drizzle of oil and pinch of salt and black pepper. Place them flat-side down on a baking sheet. Roast for 20 minutes, until soft and easily pierced with a fork.

3 Place the lentils in a medium saucepan and add water to cover by at least 2 inches (5 cm). Place over high heat, bring to a boil, then reduce the heat to medium-low and simmer for 20 minutes, until the lentils are soft. Drain and transfer to a medium bowl.

4 While the lentils cook, prepare the creamy spread by blending the goat cheese and Greek yogurt until smooth in a blender or in a bowl with a hand mixer. Set aside. In a small bowl, whisk together 1 tablespoon of the oil, the vinegar, and mustard to make the dressing. Set aside.

5 In a medium skillet, warm the remaining 1 tablespoon of oil over medium heat. Add the mushrooms, season with salt and black pepper, and cook for 3 to 5 minutes, until tender and lightly browned.

6 Pour the dressing into the bowl with the cooked lentils and mix well.

7 Divide the creamy spread among four plates. Sprinkle each with the parsley, then add the lentil salad, cooked carrots, and mushrooms. Season each salad to taste with salt and black pepper, then serve.

Pasta
with Rustic Red Lentil Marinara Sauce

+ PROTEIN + FIBER

Makes 6 to 8 servings

Pasta is a staple in many households, including mine. As much as I enjoy a classic Bolognese, meat doesn't have to be the only protein option in your pasta sauce. Incorporating red lentils to this easy marinara sauce adds protein and fiber. The red lentils cook quickly and lend a soft and delicate smoothness to this sauce, which can be used on pasta, as a pizza sauce (it's great on the Spinach and Mozzarella Pita Pizza, page 155), or in a lasagna.

---

2 tablespoons extra virgin olive oil

1 small yellow onion, diced

3 cloves garlic, minced

1 small red bell pepper, diced

2 cans (28 ounces/794 g each) whole peeled tomatoes, with juices

2 tablespoons red wine vinegar

½ cup (95 g) red lentils, rinsed and drained

1½ teaspoons dried oregano

1 teaspoon dried basil

½ teaspoon fine sea salt

1 bay leaf

Pinch crushed red pepper flakes (optional)

Black pepper

1 pound (450 g) pasta of your choice

Parmesan, grated (optional)

---

1 In a large skillet, warm the oil over medium heat. Add the onion, garlic, and bell pepper and cook until fragrant, 3 to 4 minutes. Add the tomatoes with juices, vinegar, lentils, oregano, basil, salt, bay leaf, and red pepper flakes, if using, stirring well and using the back of a wooden spoon to gently crush any large pieces of tomato. Cover, reduce the heat to low, and simmer gently for 20 to 25 minutes, until the lentils are soft and fully cooked. Remove from the heat.

2 While the sauce is simmering, bring a large pot of water to a boil. Cook the pasta according to the package instructions for al dente. Drain the pasta and divide evenly among six bowls.

3 Remove and discard the bay leaf. Use an immersion blender to puree the sauce until smooth. Season to taste with more salt, black pepper, or red pepper flakes.

4 Ladle sauce onto pasta and mix gently. Top with parmesan if using.

5 Cool any leftover sauce and store in an airtight container for up to five days in the refrigerator or three months in the freezer.

Cilantro-Lime Chicken Tacos

+ PROTEIN + FIBER

Makes 6 to 8 servings

If menopause has taught me anything, it's that flexibility is an asset. This is one of the reasons I love this chicken recipe. It shines as a weeknight meal that can be prepped ahead of time, or you can put it together from start to finish in less than 45 minutes. I like the chicken as tropical-inspired tacos topped with juicy mango, but you can use this recipe to build grain bowls, too.

½ cup (120 ml) chicken broth

Zest and juice of 3 limes, plus lime wedges for serving

2 tablespoons taco seasoning

1 tablespoon extra virgin olive oil

1 tablespoon honey

3 to 4 cloves garlic, crushed

½ teaspoon fine sea salt

1½ pounds (680 g) boneless, skinless chicken breasts

⅓ cup (20 g) roughly chopped fresh cilantro

8 soft or hard taco shells or whole wheat tortillas

1 medium carrot, finely grated or thinly sliced

1 mango, diced

1 avocado, sliced or cubed

Jalapeño slices, grated cheese, salsa, and sour cream, for topping

---

1 In a large bowl, whisk together the broth, half the lime juice and all the zest, taco seasoning, oil, honey, garlic, and salt. Place the chicken breasts in the marinade, ensuring they are fully coated. Cover and refrigerate for at least 1 hour or overnight.

2 When ready to cook, preheat the oven to 375°F (190°C).

3 Lay the chicken breasts in a shallow baking dish, along with any remaining marinade. Bake, uncovered, for 25 to 35 minutes, until the chicken has an internal temperature of 165°F (74°C).

continued

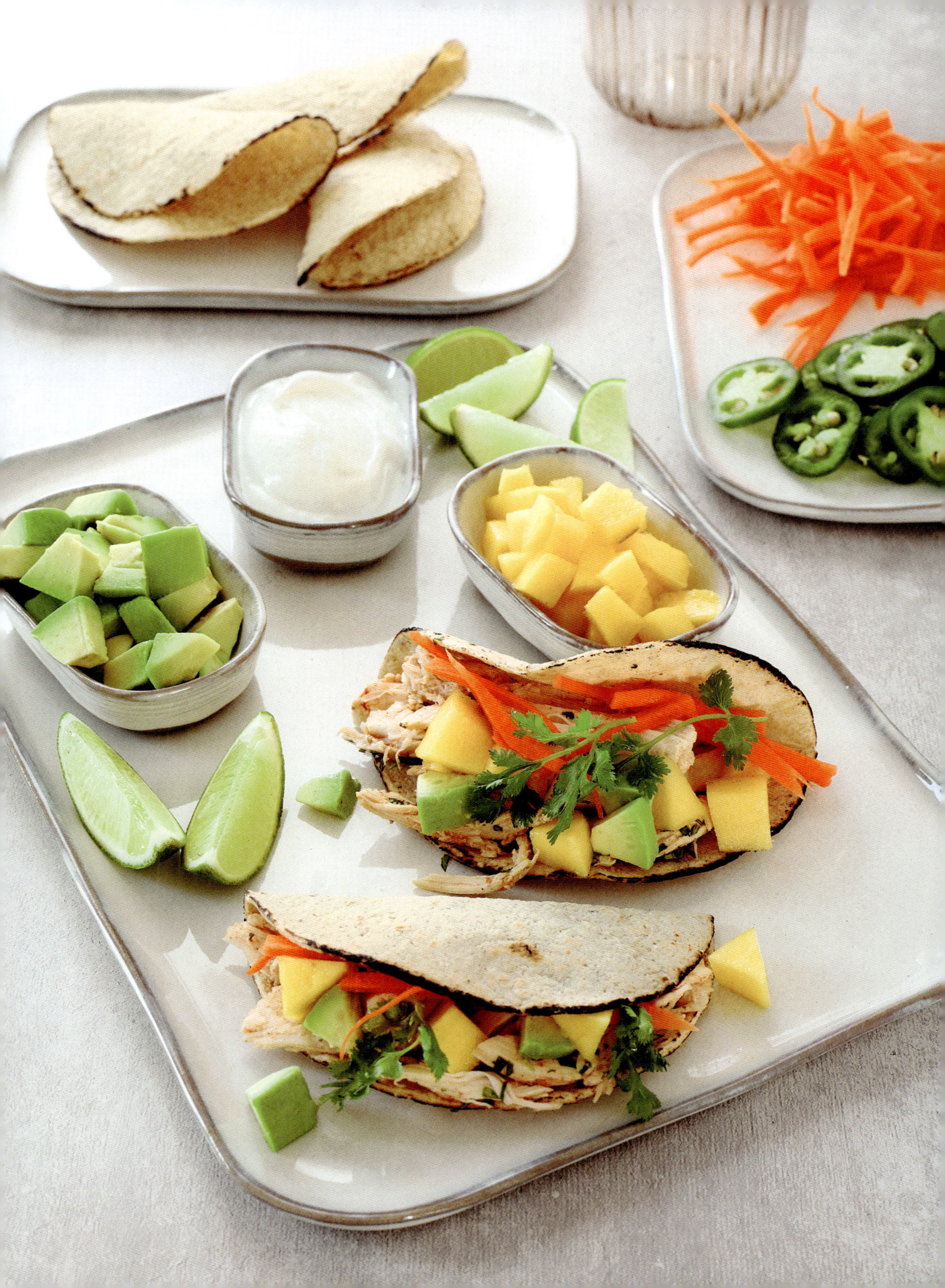

4 Transfer the chicken to a large plate. Once cooled, use two forks to shred the chicken. Mix with half of the fresh cilantro and the remaining lime juice.

5 Assemble the tacos using the shells, chicken, carrot, mango, remaining cilantro, avocado, and any other desired toppings. Serve with lime wedges on the side.

Variations

ELECTRIC PRESSURE COOKER: Use 1 cup (240 ml) chicken broth (instead of ½ cup/120 ml) and place the chicken, lime zest and juice, taco seasoning, honey, garlic, and salt in an electric pressure cooker. Cook on high pressure (or the poultry setting) for 12 minutes. Opt for the quick-release option to help keep the chicken moist. Follow steps 4 and 5 before serving.

SLOW COOKER: Combine ingredients as directed above to the electric pressure cooker and cook on low for 6 to 8 hours or high for 3 to 4 hours.

Saucy Slow-Cooked Tikka Masala

+ PROTEIN + FIBER

Makes 6 servings

If you're the kind of person who loves Indian food because of the flavorful, creamy sauces, then this recipe is for you. Tikka masala is known for its tantalizing blend of coriander, cumin, paprika, and garam masala. These spices impart a deep, earthy flavor with just a hint of smokiness from the paprika, which blends perfectly with the creamy tomato base. The nutritional yeast may seem like an unusual addition to this dish, but it adds a punch of umami that you won't regret. It also adds a dose of mood- and energy-supporting B vitamins, including vitamin B_{12}, which is a common deficiency in adults over fifty and people who follow a vegetarian diet. Both chicken and chickpeas are perfect for this recipe, and it's up to you to decide if you'll use one, the other, or both. I've used both in the instructions, but if you'd like to use one or the other, just double your chosen ingredient. Tikka masala comes together in just 30 minutes on the stovetop, but if you don't have time to supervise the cooking, throw it in a slow cooker set on low earlier in the day and walk away.

- 1½ tablespoons extra virgin olive oil
- 1 large onion, diced
- 4 cloves garlic, minced
- 1 piece (1 inch/2.5 cm) fresh ginger, minced
- 3 boneless, skinless chicken breasts, cubed
- 2 tablespoons paprika
- 1 tablespoon garam masala
- 1 teaspoon ground coriander
- 1 teaspoon ground cumin
- 1 teaspoon ground turmeric
- ½ teaspoon black pepper
- ½ teaspoon fine sea salt
- 3 tablespoons nutritional yeast
- 4 tablespoons (60 ml) tomato paste
- 1 can (14½ ounces/411 g) diced tomatoes, with juices
- 1 can (15½ ounces/439 g) chickpeas, rinsed and drained
- 1 cup (240 ml) coconut milk (reduced fat, if preferred)
- 2 tablespoons maple syrup
- Juice of 1 lemon
- 1 small bunch fresh cilantro, chopped (optional)
- Cooked rice, for serving

---

continued

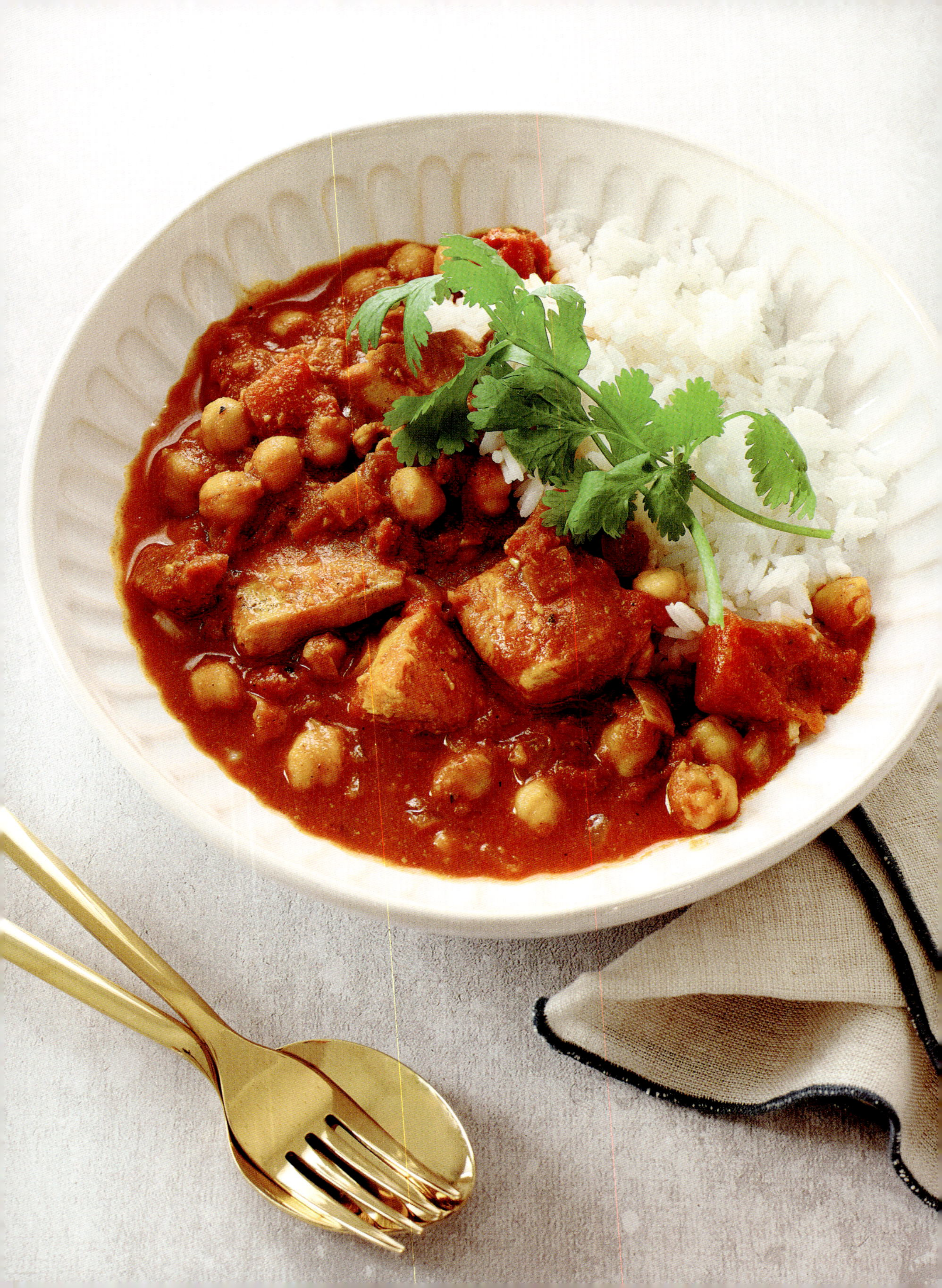

1 Warm the oil in a large pot over medium heat. Add the onion, garlic, and ginger. Cook until softened, stirring occasionally, until fragrant, 2 to 3 minutes. Add in the cubed chicken and brown on all sides, about 3 minutes, stirring occasionally to prevent sticking.

2 Add the paprika, garam masala, coriander, cumin, turmeric, black pepper, and salt. Cook the spices for 1 to 2 minutes, until fragrant. Mix in the nutritional yeast, tomato paste, and diced tomatoes (with juices), stirring well to combine. Add the chickpeas, coconut milk, and maple syrup and stir.

3 If using a slow cooker, transfer everything to the cooker and cook on low for 4 to 6 hours or on high for 2 to 3 hours. If cooking on the stovetop, cover and simmer over low heat for about 30 minutes, stirring occasionally, until the chicken is tender.

4 Just before serving, stir in the lemon juice for added brightness. Garnish with the cilantro, if using, and serve over rice.

5 Store any leftovers in an airtight container in the refrigerator for four to five days. Reheat gently on the stovetop or in the microwave, adding a splash of water or broth if needed to adjust the consistency.

Potato Chickpea Curry

+ **PROTEIN** + **FIBER**

Makes 4 servings

I grew up in potato country on the east coast of Canada, so potatoes were a big part of my life; I even attended a local potato festival every summer. It's no wonder the classic combination of potato, chickpeas, and garam masala has become my go-to comfort food now. Even though the spinach may be the last ingredient added to this dish, it brightens up your bowl while adding a big dose of heart-healthy potassium. This curry is filling on its own, but you can also serve it over rice.

---

2 teaspoons extra virgin olive oil

1 medium onion, diced

2 cloves garlic, minced, or more to taste

1½ teaspoons garam masala or 1½ tablespoons yellow curry paste, or to taste

1 teaspoon curry powder

1½ cups (350 ml) chicken or vegetable broth

1 large potato (yellow or Yukon Gold) cut into 1-inch (2.5 cm) cubes

2 cans (15½ ounces/439 g each) chickpeas, rinsed and drained

2 cups (60 g) fresh packed spinach

Fine sea salt and black pepper

Cooked rice, for serving (optional)

---

1 Warm the oil in a medium skillet over medium heat. Add the onion, garlic, garam masala, and curry powder. Cook, stirring occasionally, until fragrant, 3 to 4 minutes.

2 Add the broth and potato, reduce heat to medium-low, and simmer until the potato is just softened, about 10 minutes. Add the chickpeas and continue simmering for 5 to 10 minutes, until the potato has fully cooked. Stir in the spinach and cover the pan. Cook for 5 minutes, until the spinach has wilted.

3 Season to taste with salt and black pepper, then serve the curry on its own or over cooked rice, if using.

POTASSIUM
(IT'S IN MORE THAN JUST BANANAS)

Did you know that potassium is just as important as sodium in the heart-health conversation? It's a key ingredient in lowering blood pressure and is often lacking in our everyday diets. It's recommended that we aim for about 4,700 mg per day. You've probably heard that bananas are a good source of potassium (1 medium banana = ~440 mg), but don't forget about these other sources:

- 1 cup (180 g) cooked spinach = 840 mg
- 1 medium potato = 610 mg
- 2 wedges of watermelon = 600 mg
- 1 cup (170 g) cooked beets = 510 mg
- Half an avocado = 475 mg

Sweet Potato and Black Bean Power Bowl

+ **PROTEIN** + **FIBER**

Makes 4 servings

Here's a one-bowl meal that provides warmth and satisfaction with a side of spice and crunch. Perfect for a weeknight meal, this sweet potato and black bean rice bowl can cater to a variety of tastes. In addition to the protein and fiber provided by the beans and vegetables, the spinach and black beans also provide an impressive serving of magnesium.

---

3 medium sweet potatoes, cut into ½- to ¾-inch (12 mm to 2 cm) cubes

1 tablespoon plus ¼ cup (60 ml) extra virgin olive oil

2 teaspoons garlic powder

2 teaspoons ground cumin

¾ teaspoon fine sea salt

½ teaspoon chili powder

1 cup (185 g) uncooked long-grain rice

2 cups (475 ml) water

1 tablespoon sour cream or plain yogurt

1 teaspoon honey

Zest and juice of 1 lime, plus lime wedges for garnish

1 clove garlic, crushed

⅛ teaspoon ground cayenne pepper or paprika (optional)

Pinch of black pepper

1 can (15 ounces/425 g) black beans, rinsed and drained

1 can (15.25 ounces/432 g) corn kernels, drained

2 cups (60 g) baby spinach

1 large tomato, cubed

1 cup (110 g) shredded carrot

1 medium avocado, sliced

2 green onions, white and green parts, sliced

---

1 Preheat the oven to 375°F (190°C). Line a baking sheet with parchment paper.

2 In a large bowl, toss the sweet potatoes with 1 tablespoon of the oil, the garlic powder, cumin, ½ teaspoon of the salt, and the chili powder and spread evenly on the prepared baking sheet. Bake for 25 minutes, turning once, until the sweet potatoes are tender and a fork or knife easily slides into the center.

continued

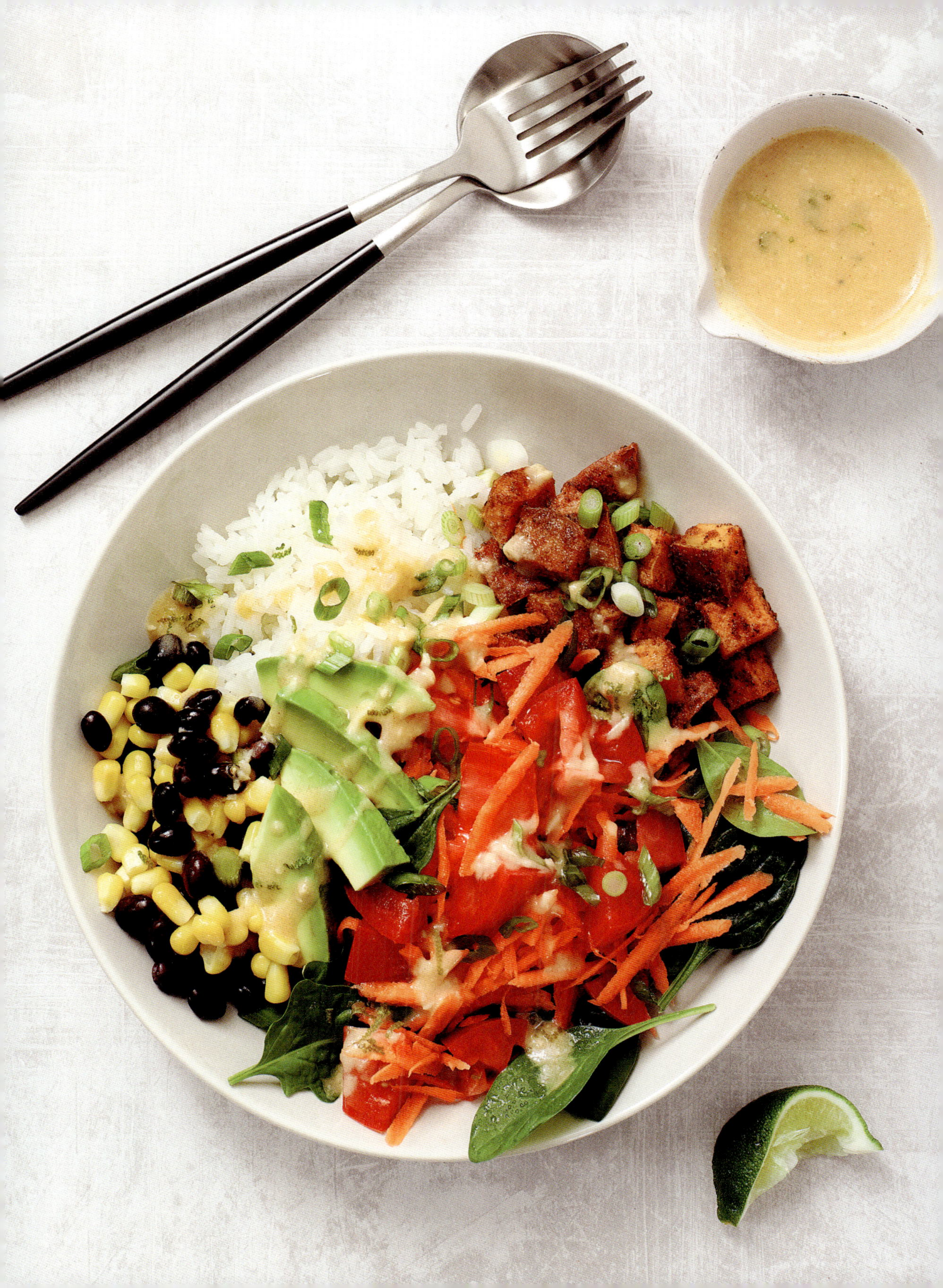

3 Meanwhile, place the rice and water in a medium pot. Bring the water to a boil over high heat, then reduce the heat to low, cover, and simmer for 15 minutes, until the water is absorbed and the rice is tender. Remove from the heat and let it sit, covered, for 5 minutes before fluffing with a fork.

4 To make the dressing, in a medium bowl, whisk together the remaining ¼ cup (60 ml) of oil, the sour cream, honey, lime zest and juice, garlic, cayenne pepper, remaining ¼ teaspoon of salt, and the black pepper.

5 Once the sweet potatoes are cooked, prepare a bowl as follows: Arrange a serving of cooked rice in one quarter of the space, the roasted sweet potatoes in the second quarter, the black beans and corn in the third quarter, and in the last quarter layer the spinach with the tomato and carrot on top. Add the avocado, sprinkle with the green onions, and drizzle with the dressing. Garnish with a wedge of lime. Repeat with the remaining ingredients for the other bowls.

Spicy Black Bean Burgers

+ PROTEIN + FIBER

Makes 8 servings

Just like a well-curated capsule wardrobe, this burger recipe is all about versatility and timeless appeal. It can fit into any meal or gathering, making it a staple for both vegetarians and meat lovers. Unlike some plant-based burgers that try too hard to be something they're not, these burgers stand confidently on their own, bringing unique flavors and texture to the table. Whether you dress them up on a classic bun or serve them as the star of a burger bowl with lettuce, tomato, and corn, reach for these when you want a protein and fiber-rich main meal.

1½ cups (350 ml) water

¾ cup (130 g) quinoa, rinsed and drained

¾ cup (75 g) rolled oats

1 can (15 ounces/425 g) black beans, rinsed and drained

2 large eggs

2 tablespoons low-sodium soy sauce or tamari

2 cloves garlic, crushed

2 teaspoons ground cumin

½ teaspoon smoked paprika

¼ teaspoon chili powder, or more to taste

¼ teaspoon ground cinnamon

¼ teaspoon fine sea salt

1 small sweet potato, cooked and mashed

2 green onions, green and white parts, finely chopped

1 to 2 teaspoons extra virgin olive oil

8 hamburger buns, toasted

Lettuce, tomato, onion, and/or cheese, for topping

---

1 In a medium saucepan, combine the water and quinoa and bring to a boil over high heat. Reduce the heat to low, cover, and simmer for 12 to 15 minutes, until the water is absorbed and the quinoa is tender. Remove from the heat and transfer the quinoa to a bowl to cool.

2 Grind ½ cup (50 g) of oats in a blender or food processor until you have a coarse flour. Transfer it to a bowl and set aside.

continued

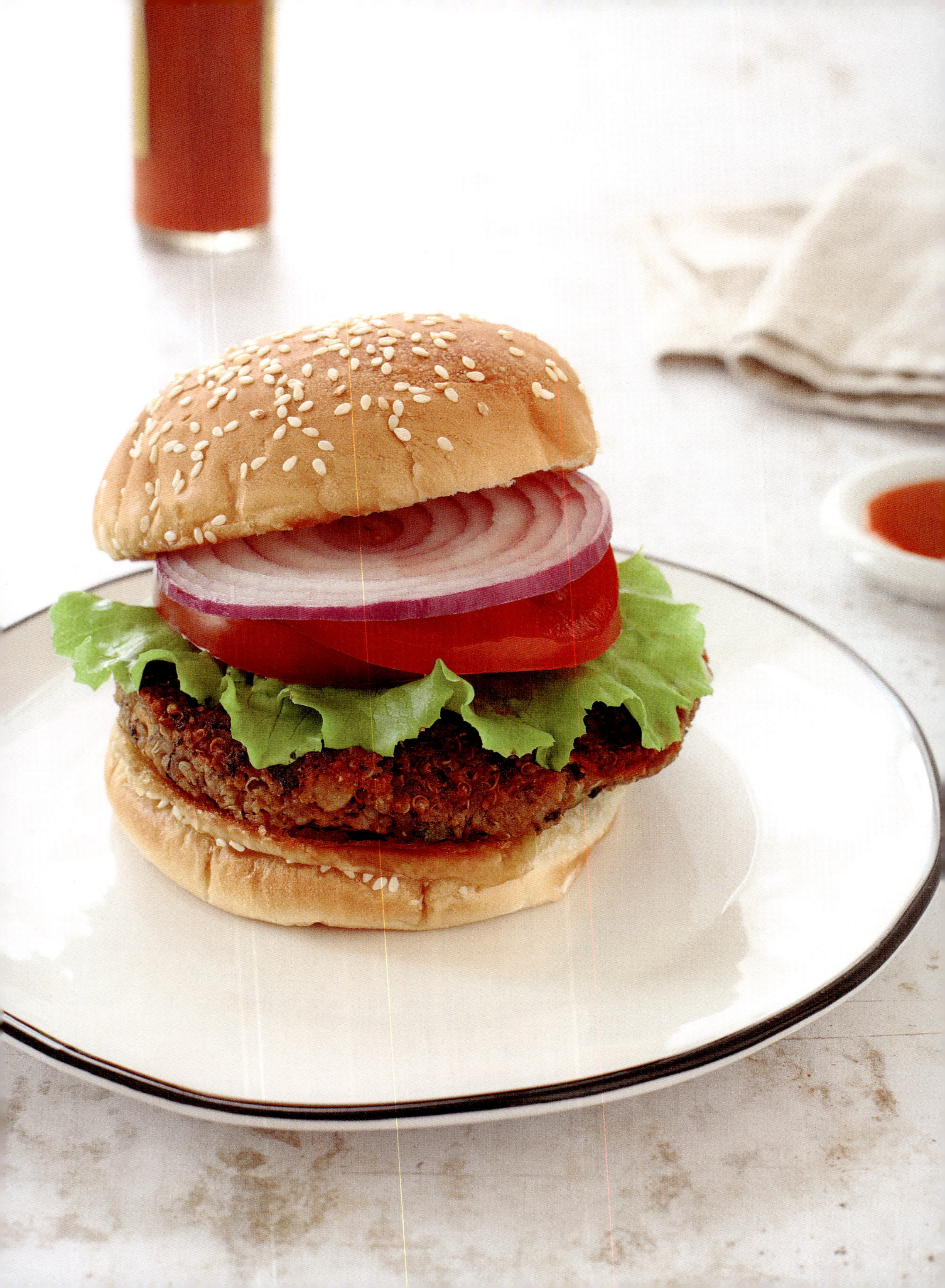

3 Combine the beans, eggs, soy sauce, garlic, cumin, paprika, chili powder, cinnamon, and salt in a food processor. Process until combined and no visible whole beans remain. Alternatively, pulse using an immersion blender. Transfer the bean mixture to a large bowl and add the cooked quinoa, sweet potato, and green onions. Mix using your hands or a fork until well combined. Stir in the ground oats and the remaining ¼ cup (25 g) of whole oats, then let the mixture sit for 10 minutes.

4 Using your hands, shape eight equal patties and set aside on a platter.

5 Warm 1 teaspoon of oil over medium heat in a large nonstick or cast-iron pan. In batches of four, cook the patties for 4 to 5 minutes per side, until lightly browned, adding more oil between batches if necessary.

6 Serve each burger on a toasted bun dressed according to your preference.

7 Cooked patties can be kept in an airtight container in the refrigerator for up to three days or in the freezer for up to six weeks.

Sheet-Pan Pistachio-Crusted Fish and Roasted Potatoes

+ PROTEIN + OMEGA-3

Makes 4 servings

Sheet-pan dinners turn weeknight meals into less of a chore. Everything roasts together on a single baking sheet, making meal prep quick—perfect if you haven't slept well or have brain fog. This recipe is incredibly versatile and works with almost any kind of fish, though salmon or halibut are my go-to choices. Pistachios add crunch and are rich in magnesium and healthy fats, while the fish provides protein and omega-3s. Serve with a side salad for a complete meal.

1¼ pounds (600 g) baby potatoes, halved

2 teaspoons extra virgin olive oil

Fine sea salt and black pepper

¾ cup (90 g) unsalted shelled roasted pistachios

¼ cup (20 g) panko breadcrumbs

1 lemon, zested and cut into wedges

1 clove garlic, minced

1½ pounds (680 g) of any skin-on fish fillet (such as halibut or salmon), cut into 4 equal pieces

3 tablespoons Dijon mustard

Fresh flat-leaf parsley, for garnish

---

1 Preheat the oven to 400°F (200°C). Line a baking sheet with parchment paper.

2 Place the potatoes in a large bowl, add the oil, a pinch each of salt and black pepper, and toss to coat. Pour the potatoes out onto the prepared baking sheet and arrange in a single layer. Put them in the oven and set a timer for 15 minutes.

3 While the potatoes roast, place the pistachios, panko, lemon zest, garlic, and a pinch each of salt and black pepper in a blender or food processor. Pulse a few times until coarsely mixed. Place the mixture in a shallow dish.

4 Prepare the fish by patting it dry and brushing the top of each piece with the mustard. Firmly press each piece of fish face down into the pistachio mixture. Place the fish on a plate.

continued

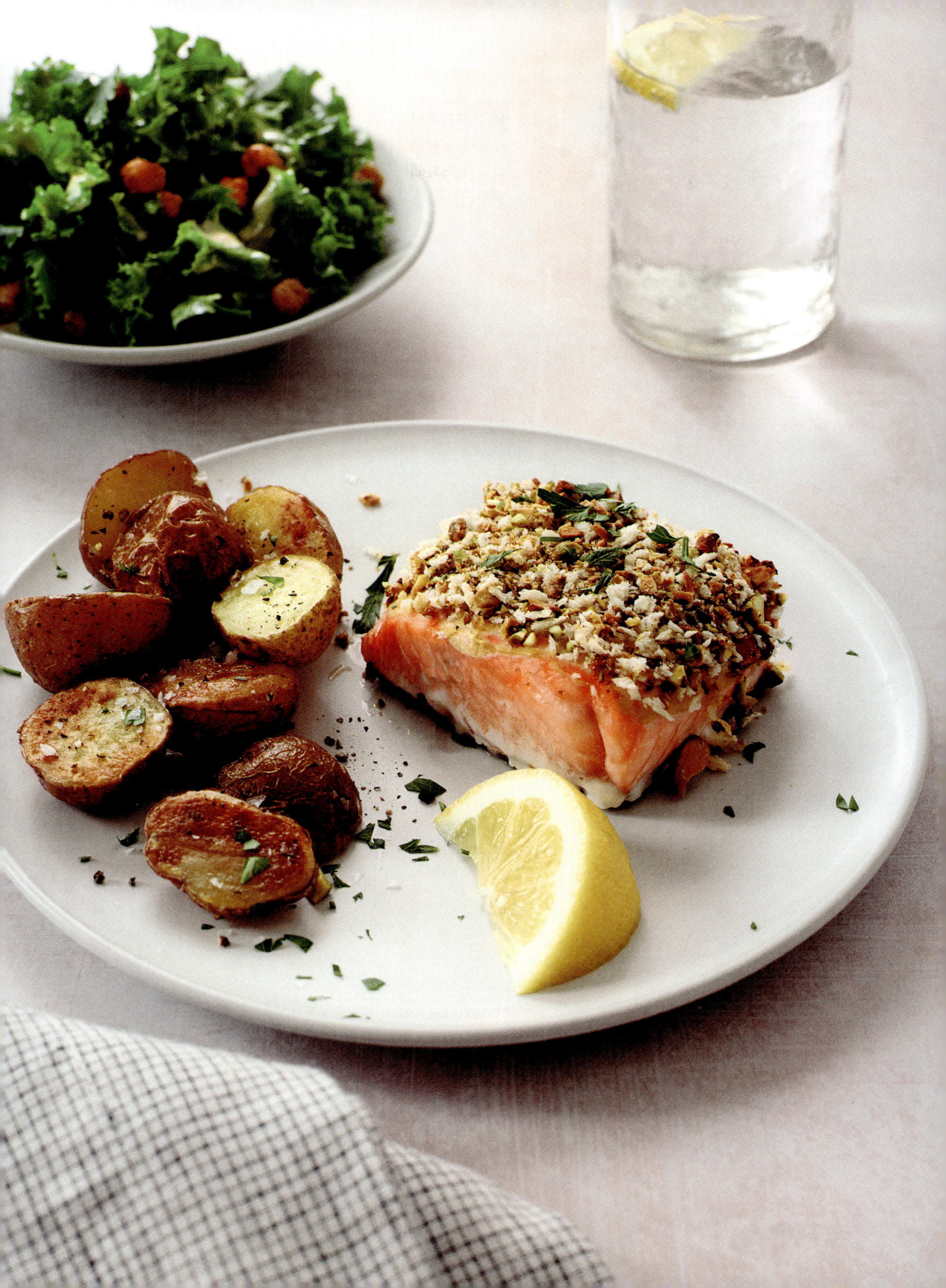

5 When the timer sounds, remove the baking sheet from the oven and stir the potatoes. Lay the fish next to the potatoes and roast 8 to 12 minutes (see note), until the potatoes are soft and easily pierced with a fork and the fish turns opaque and reaches an internal temperature of 145°F (63°C).

6 Remove from the oven and garnish with the lemon wedges and parsley before serving.

Note: When cooking fish, the rule of thumb is 10 minutes of cooking time per 1 inch (2.5 cm) of thickness, regardless of the cooking method used.

Food for Thought: Is eating fish a safe and healthy choice?

Some people avoid fish because of concerns about heavy metal contamination and sustainability. As discussed in the key ingredient section on omega-3s (page 106), there are resources you can use to make informed decisions regarding safe fishing practices. The following fish are on the FDA's list of safe fish and are excellent sources of the omega-3s EPA and DHA.

SOURCES OF OMEGA-3 FATTY ACIDS

Type of Fish	FDA Rating	EPA (mg)	DHA (mg)
Salmon, Atlantic, farmed, cooked, 3 ounces (85 g)	Best	1.24	0.59
Salmon, Atlantic, wild, cooked, 3 ounces (85 g)	Best	1.22	0.54
Herring, Atlantic, cooked, 3 ounces (85 g)	Best	0.94	0.77
Sardines, canned, 3 ounces (85 g)	Best	0.74	0.45
Halibut (Greenland), cooked, 3 ounces (85 g)	Good	0.67	0.51
Mackerel, Atlantic, cooked, 3 ounces (85 g)	Best	0.59	0.43

Data source: https://ods.od.nih.gov/factsheets/Omega3FattyAcids-HealthProfessional/.

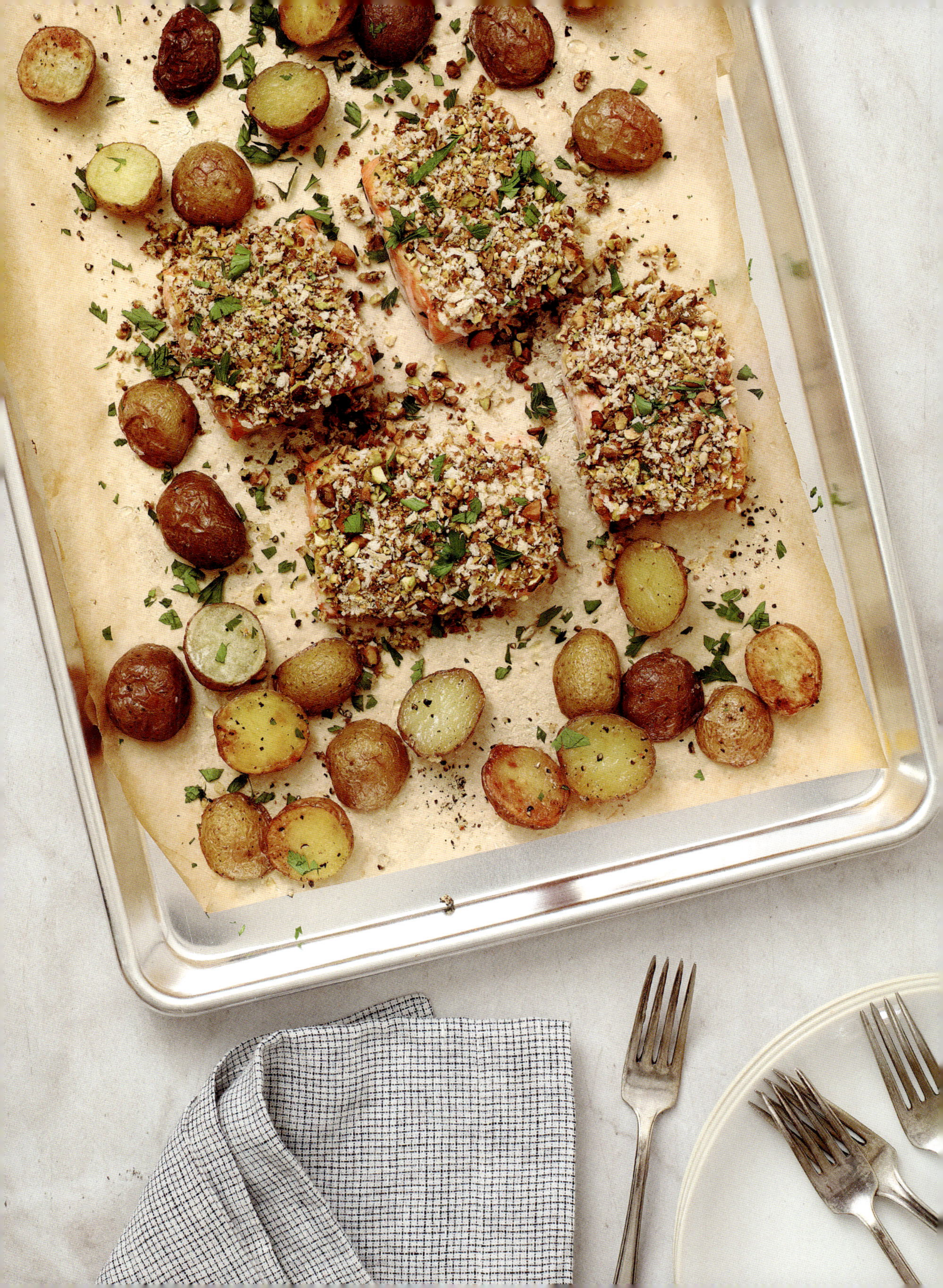

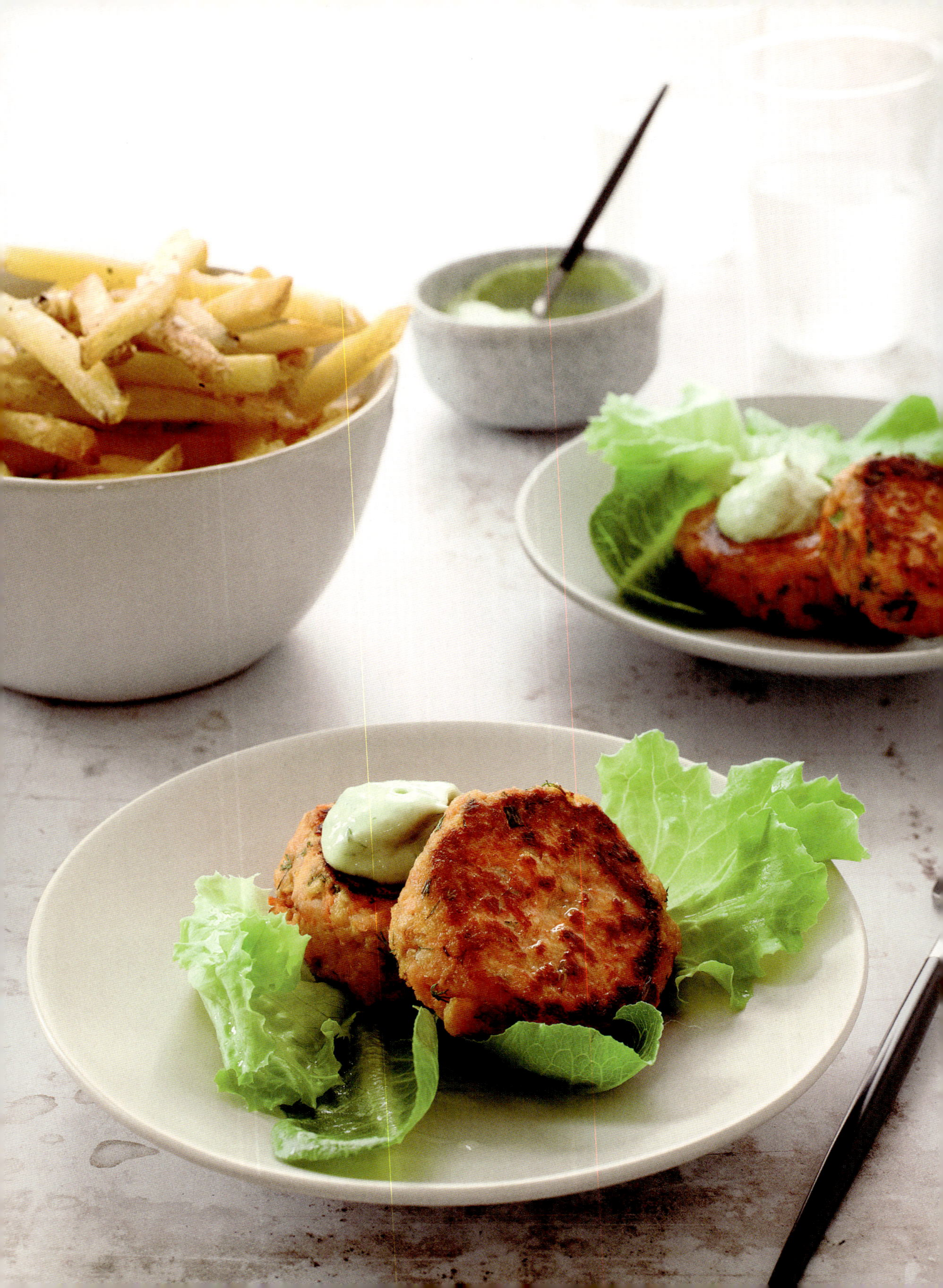

Sweet Potato Salmon Cakes

+ PROTEIN + FIBER + CALCIUM + OMEGA-3

Makes 6 cakes

Using canned salmon makes this a quick and easy meal that's full of protein, fiber, and omega-3s. Canned salmon is also an excellent source of calcium. Serve salmon cakes with a dollop of dill crema, a salad, and warmed pita bread or french fries.

- 1 medium sweet potato, peeled, cooked, and mashed
- 1 can (7½ ounces/212 g) salmon, drained
- 2 large eggs
- ¼ cup (30 g) breadcrumbs or crushed crackers, plus more as needed
- 2 tablespoons chopped fresh dill or 1 heaping teaspoon dry dill
- 1 to 2 tablespoons chopped fresh chives, to taste
- Fine sea salt and black pepper
- 2 teaspoons oil

DILL CREMA

- ½ avocado
- 3 tablespoons sour cream
- 1 tablespoon freshly squeezed lemon juice
- 2 tablespoons chopped fresh dill
- 1 clove garlic, crushed
- Pinch of salt

---

1 In a large bowl, combine the sweet potato, salmon, eggs, breadcrumbs, dill, and chives and mix well, using your hands if necessary. If the mixture is too wet to keep its shape, add more breadcrumbs, 1 tablespoon at a time. Season with salt and black pepper. Using your hands, form the mixture into six round patties and set aside on a platter.

2 Warm the oil in a large skillet over medium heat. Cook the patties for 4 to 5 minutes per side, until lightly golden.

3 To make the crema, combine the avocado, sour cream, lemon juice, dill, garlic, and salt in a blender or small food processor. Blend until smooth.

4 Serve the salmon cakes with a dollop of the crema.

Fresh and Crispy Tofu Rice Bowl

+ **SOY & PHYTOESTROGENS** + **PROTEIN** + **FIBER** + **CALCIUM**

Makes 4 servings

This crispy tofu is my kids' favorite dish that I make. Delicately crispy on the outside, soft and flavorful on the inside, crispy tofu is the perfect protein pairing for a rice bowl. Miso paste's unique flavor profile is a mix of salty, savory, and umami. It has a rich, deep taste that varies depending on the type, and white miso's mild and slightly sweet flavor pairs well with the sesame and rice vinegar in the dressing.

SUSHI RICE

1¼ cups (230 g) sushi rice

1½ cups (350 ml) cold water

5 tablespoons (75 ml) seasoned rice vinegar

Fine sea salt

TOFU

1 package (14 ounces/397 g) extra-firm tofu, drained and pressed (see page 135)

2 teaspoons sesame oil

Fine sea salt and black pepper

2 teaspoons cornstarch

1 teaspoon garlic powder

1 teaspoon onion powder

½ teaspoon paprika

½ teaspoon smoked paprika

MISO SESAME DRESSING

¼ cup (60 ml) seasoned rice vinegar

¼ cup (60 ml) water

2 tablespoons low-sodium soy sauce or tamari

1 piece (1½ inches/4 cm) fresh ginger, minced

1 clove garlic, minced

1 tablespoon white (light) miso paste

1 tablespoon sesame seeds

1 tablespoon maple syrup or honey

Zest and juice of 1 lime

2 tablespoons avocado oil

2 teaspoons sesame oil

FOR SERVING

1 mango, diced

1 avocado, diced

Baby spinach

1 medium carrot, shredded or thinly sliced

Chopped fresh cilantro

Sesame seeds

---

continued

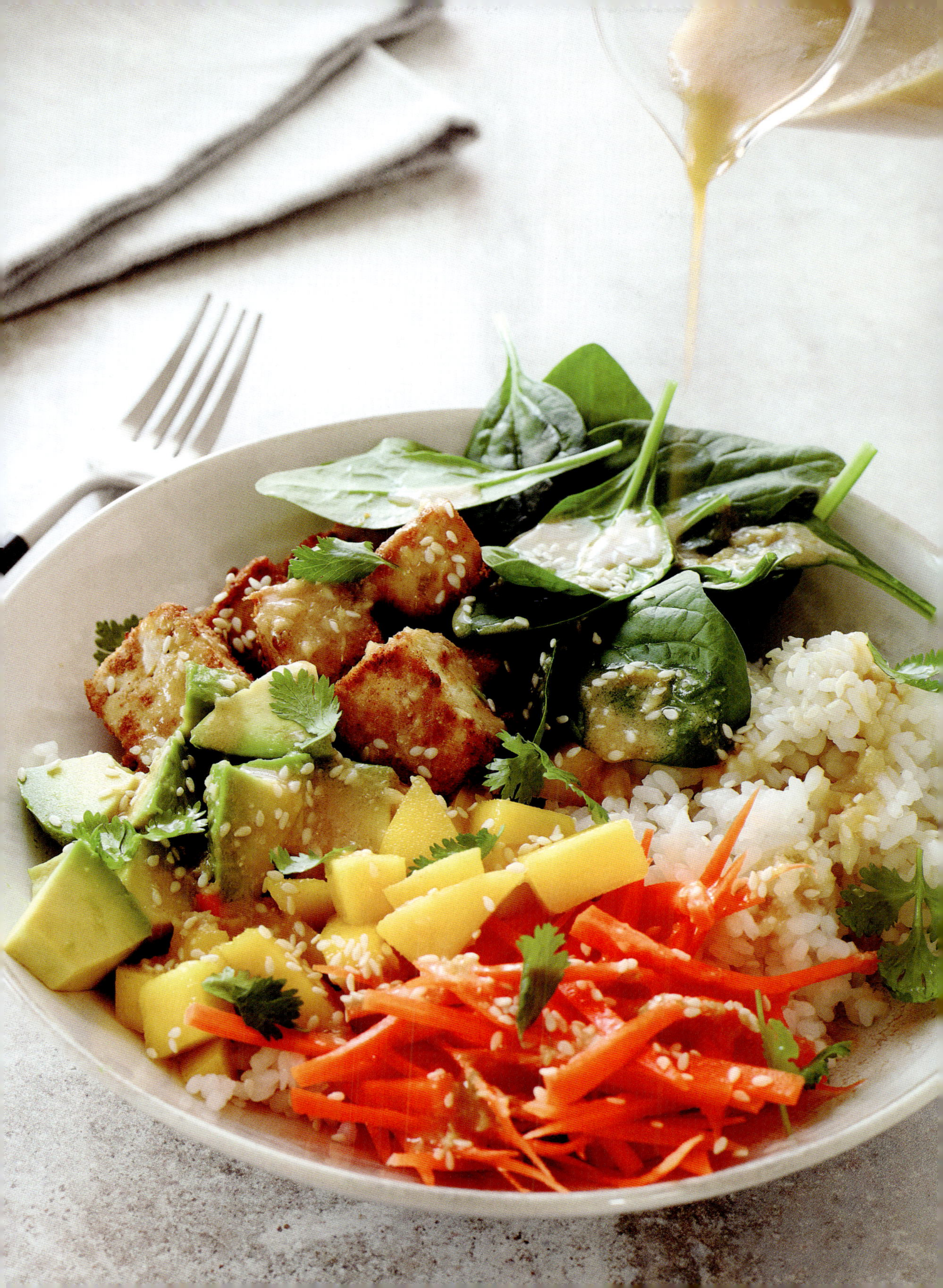

1 Preheat the oven or air fryer to 400°F (200°C). If using the oven, line a baking sheet with parchment paper.

2 To make the sushi rice, in a medium pot over high heat, bring the rice and cold water to a boil. Cover, reduce the heat to low, and simmer for 10 minutes. Remove the pot from the heat but do not uncover, then set aside for 15 minutes. In a small saucepan, heat the rice vinegar with a pinch of salt until just warm and fold it into the cooked rice. Set aside.

3 While the rice cooks and rests, prepare the tofu. Unwrap it from the paper towels and slice into equal bite-size cubes. In a large bowl, toss the tofu with the sesame oil. Season with a pinch each of salt and black pepper. In a small bowl, mix together the cornstarch, garlic powder, onion powder, paprika, and smoked paprika. Working in batches, add tofu to the cornstarch mixture, tossing the cubes gently to ensure the pieces are evenly coated.

4 To cook in the oven, place the tofu on the prepared baking sheet and bake, turning once, for 25 to 30 minutes, until lightly golden and crispy. To cook in an air fryer, place the tofu in the air fryer pan in a single layer and cook, tossing once halfway through, for 12 minutes, until lightly golden and crispy.

5 To make the miso sesame dressing, place the rice vinegar, water, soy sauce, ginger, garlic, miso paste, sesame seeds, maple syrup, and lime zest and juice in a blender. Blend for 20 to 30 seconds, until smooth. Add the avocado oil and sesame oil and blend for another 30 seconds.

6 To serve, arrange a quarter of the rice, tofu, mango, avocado, spinach, and carrots in a bowl. Add the dressing and garnish with cilantro and sesame seeds. Repeat with the remaining ingredients and serve.

Marinated Tofu and Soba Noodles with Bok Choy

+ **SOY & PHYTOESTROGENS** + **PROTEIN** + **CALCIUM**

Makes 2 to 4 servings

This nourishing dish combines tofu's phytoestrogens with nutrient-rich bok choy and satisfying soba noodles. The tofu, marinated in a savory blend of soy sauce, maple syrup, and sesame oil, pairs perfectly with the gentle crunch of bok choy and the subtle warmth of the ginger miso sauce.

MARINADE

3 tablespoons seasoned rice vinegar

2 tablespoons low-sodium soy sauce or tamari

1 tablespoon maple syrup

1 teaspoon sesame oil

2 cloves garlic, crushed

½ teaspoon ground ginger

TOFU

1 package (14 ounces/397 g) extra-firm tofu, drained and pressed (see page 135)

SAUCE

1 piece (2 inches/5 cm) fresh ginger

2 tablespoons white miso paste

1 tablespoon extra virgin olive or avocado oil

1 tablespoon seasoned rice vinegar

1 tablespoon honey

NOODLES AND BOK CHOY

8 ounces (225 g) soba noodles

2 tablespoons extra virgin olive oil

1 large head of bok choy, washed well and trimmed

Sesame seeds, for garnish

---

1 To make the marinade, in a small bowl, combine the rice vinegar, soy sauce, maple syrup, sesame oil, garlic, and ginger. Reserve 2 tablespoons of marinade for later use.

2 To prepare the tofu, pat the tofu dry and cut into 1-inch (2.5 cm) cubes. Place the cubes in a shallow dish or pan and pour the marinade over the top. Let sit for at least 30 minutes and up to 24 hours in an airtight container in the refrigerator.

continued

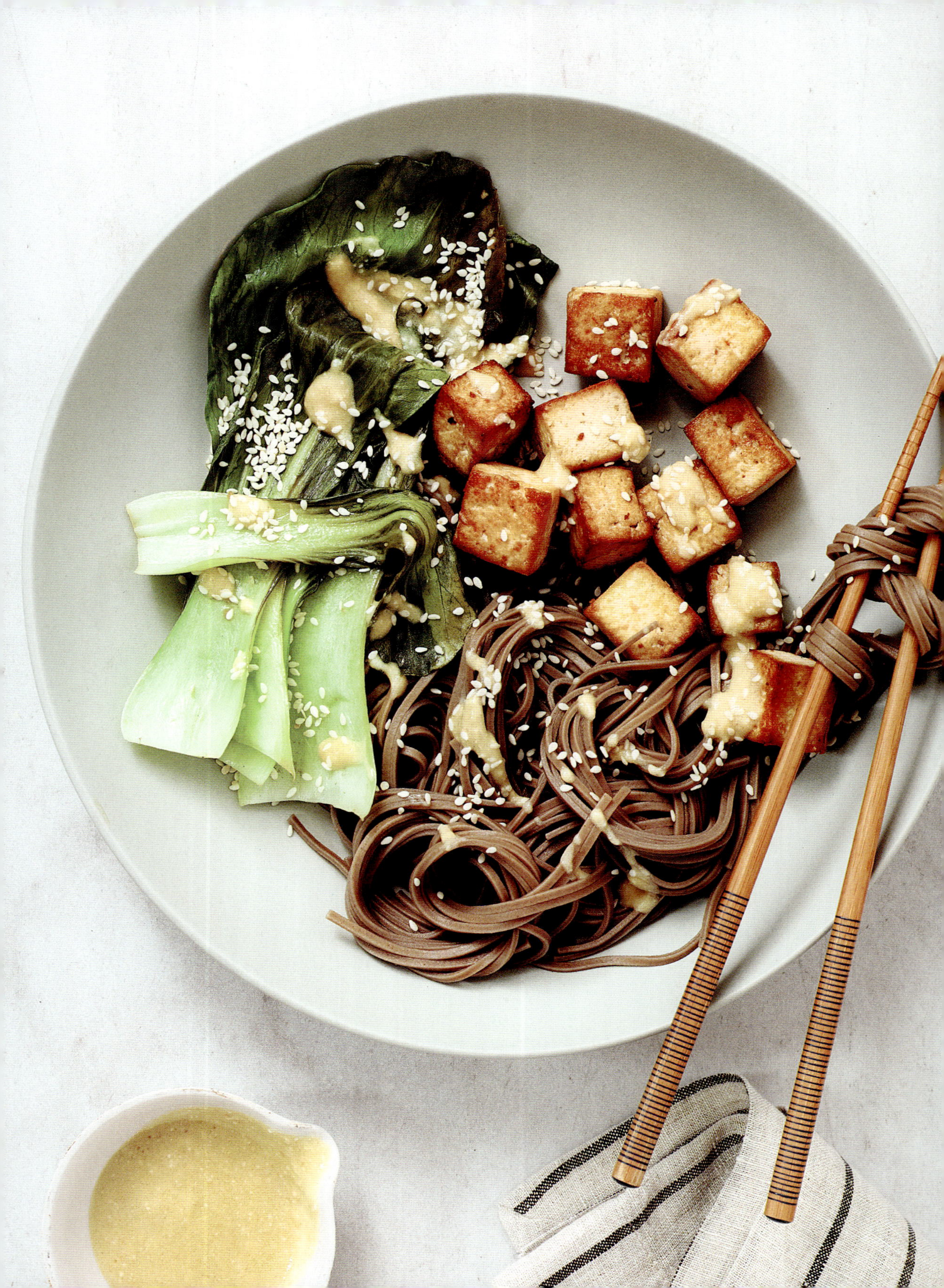

3 To make the sauce, in a small bowl, whisk together the ginger, miso paste, oil, rice vinegar, and honey. Set aside.

4 Bring a large pot of water to a boil over high heat. Reduce the heat to medium, add the soba noodles, and cook according to package instructions, usually 4 to 5 minutes. Drain and rinse the noodles under cold water to cool. Set aside in a large bowl.

5 While you wait for the water to boil, warm the olive oil in a large cast-iron skillet over medium heat. Using a slotted spoon, transfer the tofu from the marinade to the skillet in a single layer. Cook, turning occasionally, until golden brown on all sides, 8 to 12 minutes.

6 Remove the tofu from the skillet and set aside on a plate. Pour the reserved marinade into the same skillet and add the boy choy. Cook the bok choy for 3 to 5 minutes, until the leafy green parts are wilted and a fork easily pierces the white stems.

7 Transfer the noodles, cooked tofu, and bok choy to plates, drizzle the sauce over the top, garnish with sesame seeds, and serve.

Variation

MARINATED SHRIMP: If you'd like to try the dish with something other than tofu, you can easily use 1 pound (450 g) of shrimp instead. Buy fresh or frozen *raw* peeled shrimp as it soaks up the flavors of the marinade more easily, but cooked shrimp can work in a pinch.

Salads and Small Plates

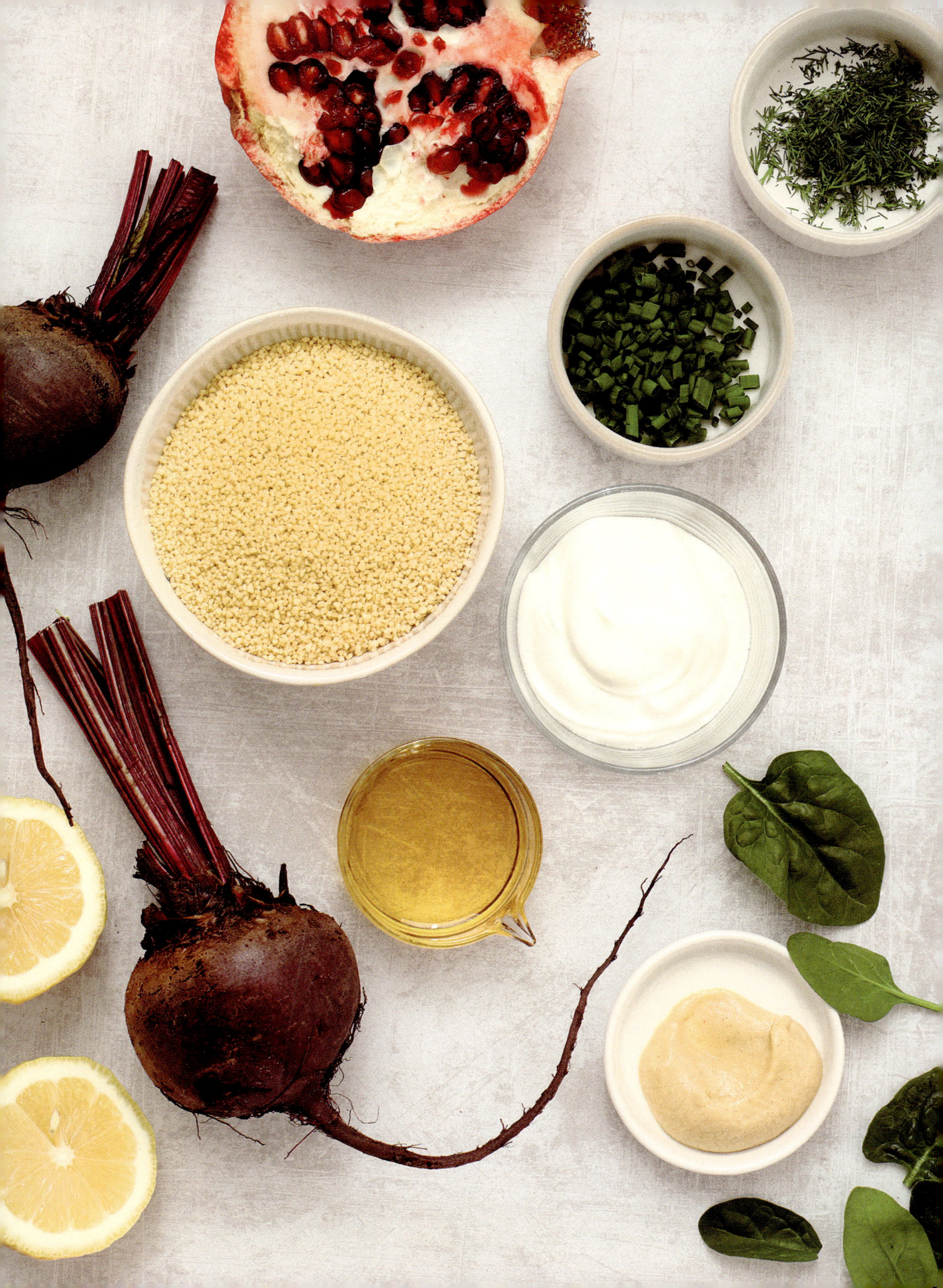

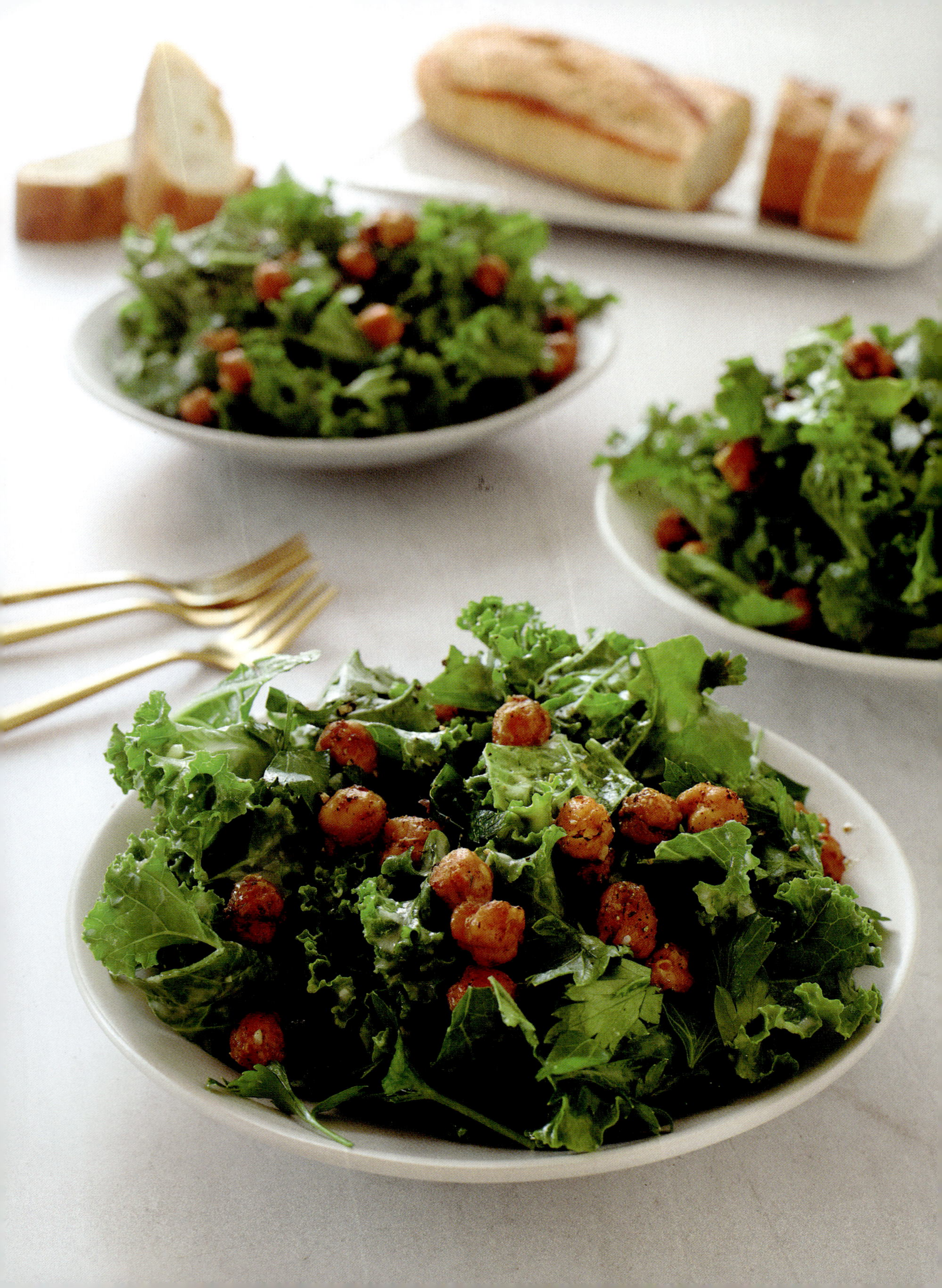

Lemon Lovers Creamy Kale Salad with Roasted Chickpeas

+ PROTEIN + FIBER + CALCIUM

Makes 4 servings

Lemon, garlic, and tahini are a classic trio of flavors. But it's the roasted chickpeas marinated in a lemony spice blend that make this salad a standout. As a low-oxalate leafy green vegetable, kale has calcium that is more easily absorbed compared to other greens like spinach. When paired with the tahini, this salad gives you a substantial deposit in your calcium bank!

---

1 can (15½ ounces/439 g) chickpeas, rinsed and drained

2 tablespoons extra virgin olive oil

Juice of 3 small lemons, plus more for squeezing

Zest of 1 small lemon

1 teaspoon garlic powder

1 teaspoon ground turmeric

1 teaspoon paprika

Fine sea salt and black pepper

1 large bunch curly kale

¼ cup (60 g) tahini

1 tablespoon honey

2 cloves garlic, peeled

2 to 4 tablespoons (30 to 60 ml) hot water

Chopped fresh flat-leaf parsley, for serving

Fresh baguette, for serving

---

1 Preheat the oven to 400°F (200°C). Line a baking sheet with parchment paper.

2 Blot the chickpeas dry with a towel. This essential step helps the chickpeas soak up the flavor of the lemon and spices. In a medium bowl, toss the chickpeas with 1 tablespoon of the oil, 1½ tablespoons of lemon juice, the lemon zest, garlic, turmeric, paprika, and a pinch each of salt and black pepper. Coat evenly.

3 Spread the chickpeas in a single layer on the prepared baking sheet and bake for 30 minutes, until lightly golden but still soft, shaking and turning the pan after 15 minutes. Allow the chickpeas to cool.

continued

4 Prepare the kale by removing the leaves from the stems (you can discard the tough stems). Wash and rinse the leaves under cold water and tear the greens into bite-size pieces. Place the kale in a large bowl and add the remaining 1 tablespoon of oil. Using your hands, massage the kale pieces with the oil. This will make the kale tender and soft. Set aside.

5 Prepare the dressing by combining the tahini, remaining lemon juice, honey, garlic, salt, black pepper, and 2 tablespoons of the hot water in a blender. Blend until smooth. If the dressing is too thick, add 1 tablespoon of hot water at a time until it reaches the desired consistency.

6 Add about half of the dressing to the kale and stir to coat evenly. Add the remaining dressing, 1 to 2 tablespoons at a time, until the salad is as creamy as you like it.

7 Mix in the roasted chickpeas, then finish with a squeeze of fresh lemon juice and parsley. Serve immediately with the baguette.

Undiet It! Going Green

Leafy greens pack a lot of nutrient density into their leaves, and some of them, such as kale, took on superfood status in the early 2000s. It's easy to get caught up in the race for good, better, and best. But if we assume that all plants "count," we can lead with satisfaction when choosing which leafy green to munch on.

I like using kale in this salad as it holds its shape and crisp texture when mixed with a creamy sauce and roasted chickpeas. As a cooked green, I don't enjoy its chewy texture. When I want a crispy and crunchy green, I lead toward romaine lettuce or Boston Bibb lettuce. Softer greens like spinach and Swiss chard are good go-to greens in warm dishes. Notice that I don't choose my greens based on nutrition but rather taste and texture? That's how to lead with satisfaction!

Warm and Tangy Winter Kale Salad

+ PROTEIN + FIBER + CALCIUM

Makes 2 to 4 servings

Despite the year-round hot flash forecast, you might shy away from salads when the weather cools off. But this warm and tangy salad with lightly sauteed kale provides just the right amount of warmth. Kale is well-suited to colder days, and I've known many people who keep it growing in their garden well into winter. Your body and bones will appreciate the protein, fiber, and calcium from the kale, tahini, and chickpeas. This can be enjoyed on its own or as a side to a chicken or fish dish.

---

2 teaspoons plus 1 tablespoon extra virgin olive oil

1 small bunch lacinato kale or other variety, torn into bite-size pieces

½ red bell pepper, sliced

½ yellow bell pepper, sliced

1 can (15½ ounces/439 g) chickpeas, rinsed and drained

½ cup (90 g) diced cherry tomatoes

2 to 4 tablespoons (18 to 36 g) nutritional yeast (more if you like it tangy, less for a more subtle taste)

2 tablespoons tahini

1 to 2 cloves garlic, peeled

Juice of 1 lemon

¼ teaspoon salt

1 tablespoon water, plus more as needed

½ cup (75 g) diced cucumber

2 tablespoons chopped pecans

---

1 Warm 2 teaspoons of the oil in a medium skillet over medium heat. Add the kale and red and yellow bell peppers and cook, stirring occasionally, for 2 to 3 minutes, until just softened.

2 Add the chickpeas and tomatoes and cook for 2 to 4 minutes, stirring gently to ensure even cooking. The tomatoes should begin to soften and release some juices but still hold their shape. Remove from the heat and set aside.

continued

3 Prepare the dressing by combining the nutritional yeast, tahini, the remaining 1 tablespoon of oil, the garlic, lemon juice, and salt in a blender or food processor. Blend until smooth. Add the water, a little at a time, until the dressing has a pourable consistency.

4 Transfer the chickpeas and kale mixture to a medium bowl. Gently mix in half of the dressing until evenly coated. Add the cucumbers and pecans just before serving. Drizzle with remaining dressing and enjoy.

Feast on This!

Nutritional yeast is a deactivated yeast (*Saccharomyces cerevisiae*) that's known for its savory, cheese-like flavor. Unlike the yeast used for baking or brewing, nutritional yeast is nonleavening, meaning it doesn't cause dough to rise or ferment beverages. It originally gained popularity among vegans and vegetarians as a cheese substitute, but its unique umami taste gives it broader appeal. Rich in energy-supporting B vitamins, including B_{12}, it's a great addition to your menopause kitchen. It's also delicious sprinkled on hot popcorn, so you don't need to worry about it going to waste in your pantry.

Tofu Broccoli Salad
with Kimchi Miso Dressing

+ **SOY & PHYTOESTROGENS** + **PROTEIN** + **FIBER** + **CALCIUM**

Makes 2 to 4 servings

Some people may be intimidated by cooking tofu or find its texture unfamiliar, but once you learn the secret to making perfect tofu, it'll become one of your staple ingredients. Crispy tofu is the ideal pairing to this crunchy salad. Kimchi adds a kick of spice in the dressing, along with a dose of gut-loving probiotics.

TOFU

1 package (14 ounces/397 g) extra-firm tofu (see page 135)

1 tablespoon seasoned rice vinegar

1 tablespoon toasted sesame oil

1 tablespoon soy sauce or tamari

1 teaspoon honey

1 tablespoon cornstarch

1 teaspoon garlic powder

1 teaspoon ground ginger

½ teaspoon ground cumin

½ teaspoon ground coriander

Pinch of cayenne pepper (optional)

DRESSING

⅓ cup water

¼ cup (45 g) kimchi

2 tablespoons extra virgin olive oil

1 tablespoon toasted sesame oil

1 tablespoon seasoned rice vinegar

2 teaspoons white or red miso paste

2 teaspoons honey

SALAD

1 large head of broccoli, cut into small florets

1 large carrot, grated

½ cup (80 g) diced red onion

⅔ cup (90 g) roasted unsalted sunflower seeds

1 or 2 small green onion tops, chopped

---

continued

1 Preheat the oven to 425°F (220°C). Line a baking sheet with parchment paper.

2 To prepare the tofu, drain it and squeeze out as much water as possible by pressing it firmly between your hands. Wrap the tofu in a tea towel or paper towels and place it on a plate. Place a heavy pan on top and let it drain for at least 15 minutes. Cut the tofu into 1-inch (2.5 cm) cubes and set aside.

3 Whisk the vinegar, sesame oil, soy sauce, and honey in a medium bowl until well combined. Add the tofu to the bowl and toss lightly to coat. Marinate for at least 15 minutes or up to overnight, in an airtight container in the refrigerator, for better flavor.

4 Place the cornstarch, garlic powder, ginger, cumin, coriander, and cayenne pepper, if using, in a medium bowl and mix well, ensuring that no clumps are visible. Transfer the tofu to the cornstarch mixture, tossing the cubes gently to ensure the pieces are evenly coated.

5 Spread the tofu in an even layer on the prepared baking sheet. Cook for 15 minutes, then flip the tofu and cook for another 10 to 15 minutes, until lightly golden and crispy.

6 Meanwhile, make the dressing. Combine the water, kimchi, olive oil, sesame oil, rice vinegar, miso paste, and honey in a blender. Blend until smooth.

7 To make the salad, place the broccoli, carrot, onion, and half of the dressing in a large bowl. Toss until evenly coated. Add the tofu and sunflower seeds along with the remainder of the dressing. Toss and top with green onions before serving.

Note: The tofu can also be cooked in an air fryer. Preheat an air fryer to 400°F (200°C) and arrange the tofu in a single layer and cook for 12 to 14 minutes, until lightly golden and crispy, tossing once halfway through cooking.

Smashed Chickpea Salad

+ PROTEIN + FIBER

Makes 2 to 4 servings

Cook once and eat twice is one of my favorite mottos. And there's nothing I love more than a recipe with leftovers *and* some built-in flexibility. Chickpeas are the star of this simple salad that can be enjoyed with pasta or as a wrap (see variation). Packed with protein, fiber, and crunch, this salad is an all-around winner.

¾ cup (150 g) orzo pasta

2 teaspoons Dijon mustard

1 teaspoon apple cider vinegar

1 teaspoon extra virgin olive oil

Zest and juice of 1 lemon

Fine sea salt and black pepper

1 can (15½ ounces/439 g) chickpeas, rinsed and drained

2 tablespoons finely chopped red onion

1 tablespoon chopped fresh flat-leaf parsley

½ cup (75 g) diced cucumber

1 avocado, sliced (optional)

1 Fill a medium pot with water, place it over high heat, and bring to a boil. Add the pasta and cook according to the package instructions. Drain the pasta and allow to cool for 15 minutes.

2 In a large bowl, whisk together the mustard, vinegar, oil, and lemon juice and zest, then season to taste with salt and black pepper. Add the chickpeas and mix gently until they are evenly coated with the dressing. Using the back of a large spoon or fork, gently crush the chickpeas until most have a smashed appearance but are not fully mashed.

3 Add the onion, parsley, and cucumber and mix well. Fold the cooked pasta into the chickpea salad until evenly combined. Top with avocado, if using, just before serving

Variation

CHICKPEA WRAPS: Omit the pasta and finely dice the cucumber for easier folding. Spoon some of the chickpea salad into a tortilla wrap and top with sliced avocado, if using.

Cilantro Black Bean Salad

+ PROTEIN + FIBER

Makes 2 to 4 servings

Don't judge a book by its cover, and don't judge a recipe by its simplicity. This fresh and simple salad can hold its own as a meal but also plays well with others. I like to serve black bean salad alongside chicken or shrimp skewers cooked on the grill. The salad also makes for a quick and easy taco filling—just add your favorite taco seasoning.

- 1 can (15 ounces/425 g) black beans, rinsed and drained
- 1 large handful fresh cilantro, roughly chopped
- 1 avocado, cubed (see note)
- 1 large tomato, diced
- ½ cup (85 g) fresh or frozen corn kernels
- 1 small cucumber, diced
- 1 red bell pepper, diced
- 1 tablespoon extra virgin olive oil
- Juice of 1 lime
- 1 clove garlic, minced
- Fine sea salt and black pepper

---

1 In a large bowl, combine the black beans, cilantro, avocado, tomato, corn, cucumber, and bell pepper. Gently toss the ingredients to mix evenly.

2 In a small bowl, whisk together the oil, lime juice, and garlic. Season to taste with salt and black pepper. Drizzle this dressing over the salad and toss again to ensure all the ingredients are well coated.

3 Allow the salad to chill in the refrigerator for about 30 minutes before serving. This step helps enhance the flavors, but if you're short on time, you can serve it immediately.

Note: If you're making this salad more than 30 minutes before serving, hold off on adding the avocado until you're ready to eat.

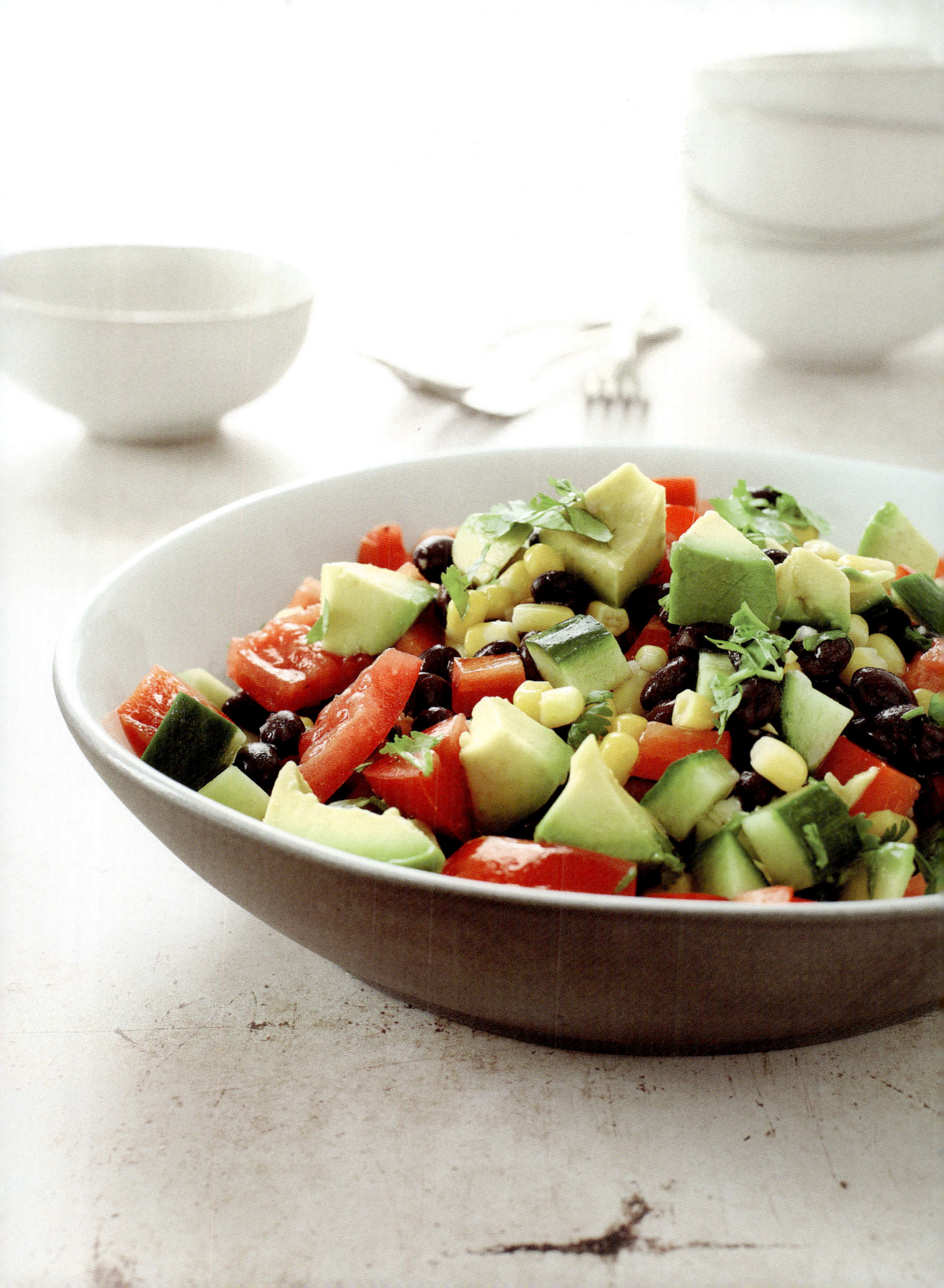

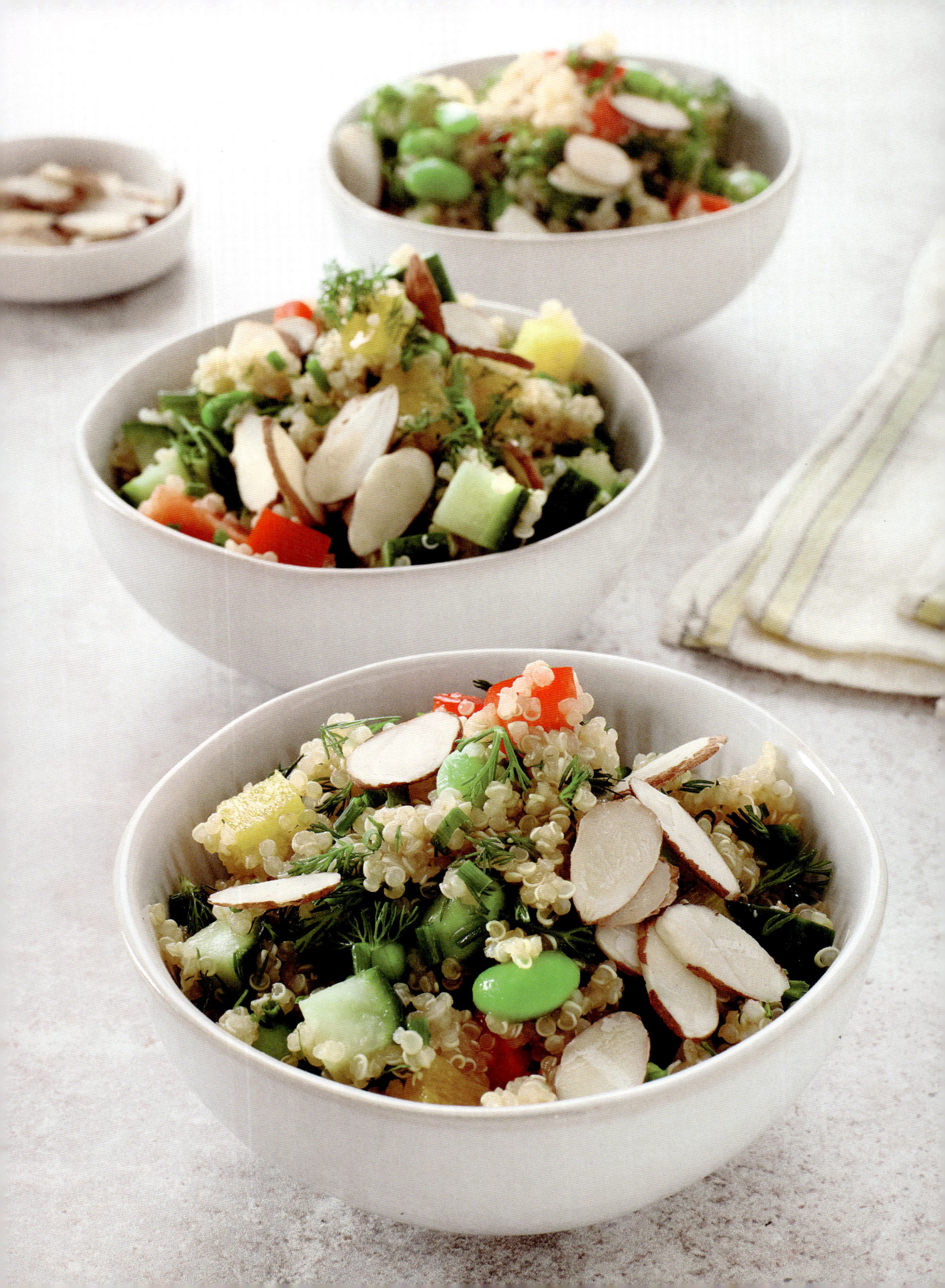

Easy Edamame, Dill, and Quinoa Salad

+ SOY & PHYTOESTROGENS + PROTEIN + FIBER

Makes 4 to 6 servings

My favorite time of the year is when the farmers market starts overflowing with fresh herbs, including my favorite, fresh dill. The familiar flavors of dill and cucumber come together perfectly in this dish that can be enjoyed on its own or as a side. Edamame adds an impressive serving of phytoestrogens, protein, and fiber that will help keep you full for hours.

---

2 cups (475 ml) vegetable broth

1 cup (170 g) white quinoa, rinsed and drained

3 tablespoons apple cider or white vinegar

2 tablespoons extra virgin olive oil

½ teaspoon fine sea salt

1 cup (160 g) cooked shelled edamame, cooled

1 medium cucumber, diced

½ cup (75 g) diced red bell pepper

½ cup (75 g) diced yellow bell pepper

⅓ cup (20 g) roughly chopped fresh dill

⅓ cup (15 g) thinly sliced fresh chives

Black pepper

⅓ cup (30 g) sliced almonds (optional)

---

1 Pour the broth into a medium saucepan and bring it to a boil over high heat. Add the quinoa, reduce the heat to low, cover, and simmer for 15 minutes, until all the water is absorbed and the quinoa is soft and fluffy. Set aside to cool for 30 minutes.

2 Whisk together the vinegar, oil, and salt in a large bowl. Mix in the cooked quinoa, edamame, cucumber, red and yellow bell peppers, dill, and chives. Season to taste with salt and black pepper.

3 Top with sliced almonds, if using, and serve immediately.

4 Store in an airtight container in the refrigerator for up to five days.

So Easy Soba Noodle Salad

+ SOY & PHYTOESTROGENS + PROTEIN + FIBER

Makes 4 servings

This soba noodle salad topped with a peanut-ginger dressing is a great make-ahead meal that tastes even better the next day. You can enjoy it warm, but I prefer it cold—especially during the warm weather months. The combination of crunchy vegetables, tender soba noodles, and a tangy, nutty dressing will leave you feeling refreshed and nourished.

8 ounces (225 g) soba noodles

⅓ cup (95 g) natural peanut butter

2 tablespoons reduced-sodium soy sauce

2 tablespoons rice vinegar

1 tablespoon sesame oil

1 tablespoon water, plus more as needed

1 tablespoon honey

Juice of 1 lime, plus lime wedges for serving

1 piece (1 inch/2.5 cm) fresh ginger, grated

1 large clove garlic, minced

2 cups (125 g) whole sugar snap peas, halved diagonally

1 red bell pepper, thinly sliced

1 cup (160 g) shelled edamame

1 medium carrot, grated or thinly sliced

1 tablespoon white or black sesame seeds

---

1 Bring a large pot of water to a boil over high heat. Reduce the heat to medium, add the soba noodles, and cook according to package instructions, usually 4 to 5 minutes. Drain and rinse the noodles under cold water to cool. Set aside in a large bowl.

2 In a small bowl, whisk together the peanut butter, soy sauce, vinegar, sesame oil, 1 tablespoon of water, honey, lime juice, ginger, and garlic until smooth. If the mixture is too thick, add 1 tablespoon of water at a time until it reaches a pourable consistency.

3 Gently fold half of the dressing into the bowl with the cooked soba noodles until evenly coated. Add the snap peas, bell pepper, edamame, and carrot and drizzle with the remaining dressing. Top with sesame seeds and serve with a wedge of lime. Serve immediately for a warm noodle salad or refrigerate for 1 to 2 hours if serving as a cold dish.

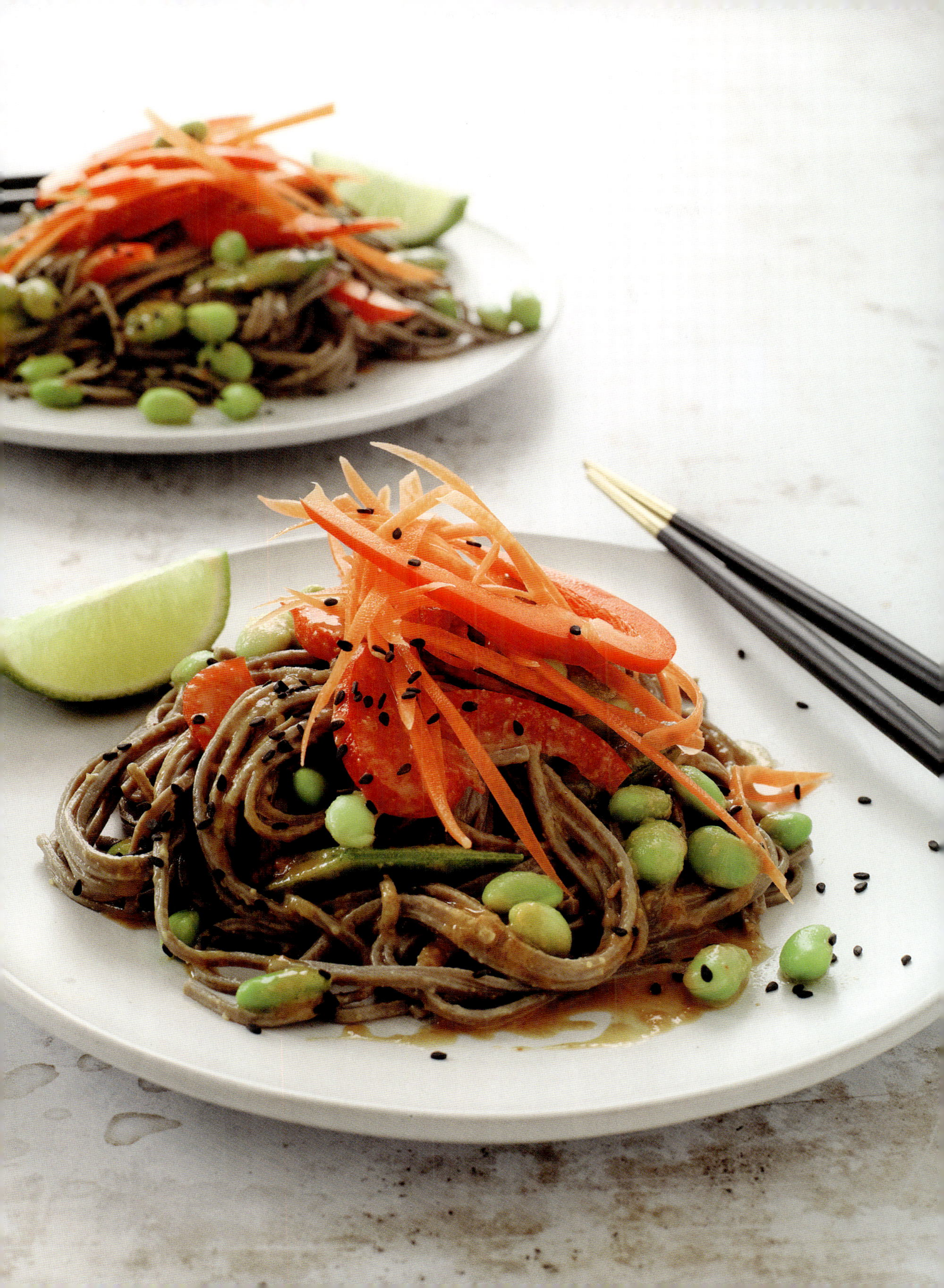

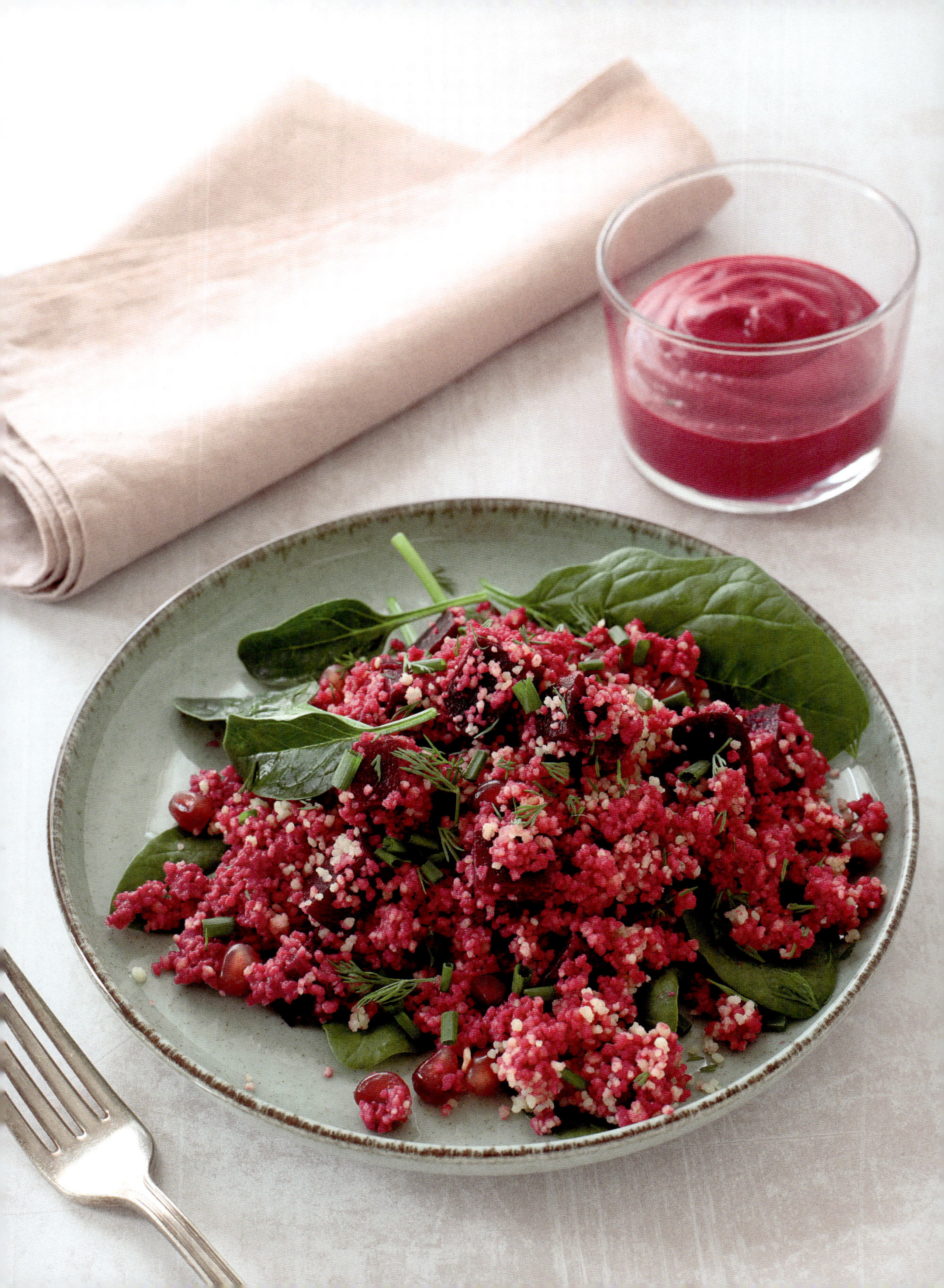

Beet and Pomegranate Couscous

+ **FIBER**

Makes 2 to 4 servings

Beets brighten up any dish with both color and flavor. Along with spinach, beets are also an excellent source of heart-healthy potassium.

---

3 medium beets

1 cup (170 g) couscous

⅔ cup (160 ml) boiling water

¼ cup (60 g) plain Greek yogurt

Zest and juice of 1 lemon

1 tablespoon extra virgin olive oil

1 tablespoon water

½ teaspoon Dijon mustard

1 pomegranate

6 ounces (170 g) baby spinach

3 tablespoons chopped fresh dill

3 tablespoons chopped fresh chives

---

1 Rinse the beets under cold water. Halve each beet and place in a medium pot, cover with water, and bring to a boil over high heat. Reduce the heat to medium-low and simmer for 30 minutes, until tender. Transfer the beets to a dish, cover, and cool for 10 minutes. Gently rub off the skins with your hands or a paper towel and discard. Set the beets aside.

2 Place the couscous in a large bowl and add the boiling water. Mix with a fork, cover, and set aside for 15 minutes.

3 To make the dressing, combine 4 of the cooked beet halves, the yogurt, lemon zest and juice, oil, the 1 tablespoon water, and the mustard in a blender or food processor and blend until smooth.

4 Slice the remaining beet halves into small cubes and set aside.

5 Halve the pomegranate and hold a section over a bowl, seed-side down. Firmly tap the pomegranate with the back of a wooden spoon to release the seeds. Repeat with the other half.

6 Fluff the couscous with a fork and mix in some of the dressing. Stir in the beets and pomegranate seeds. Layer the spinach and couscous on a plate, adding more dressing. Sprinkle with the dill and chives before serving.

Tuna Salad with Cranberry

+ PROTEIN + OMEGA-3

Makes 2 servings

Tuna may be a lunchtime staple, but that doesn't mean it has to be boring. Crunchy foods bring so much pleasure to our palate, as do the pops of sweetness from the dried cranberries. I often eat this salad as part of a bento box lunch and spoon it onto crackers and sliced cucumbers, but you could enjoy it as a sandwich, too. A balanced midday meal can help ward off afternoon brain fog and keep your energy stable until dinner. You can easily double or triple this recipe and store in a covered dish in the refrigerator for up to three days.

---

2 tablespoons mayonnaise

1 tablespoon freshly squeezed lemon juice (about ½ lemon)

1 can (5 ounces/142 g) tuna in water, drained

⅓ cup (30 g) diced celery

2 tablespoons dried cranberries

2 tablespoons diced red onion

Fine sea salt and black pepper

Crackers or bread, for serving

---

1 In a medium bowl, whisk together the mayonnaise and lemon juice until smooth. Flake the tuna into the bowl. Add the celery, cranberries, and onion. Mix well using a large fork or spoon before seasoning to taste with salt and black pepper.

2 For best flavor, refrigerate the tuna salad for about 30 minutes before serving on crackers or as a sandwich.

Roasted Vegetables
with Tangy Miso Dressing

+ **SOY & PHYTOESTROGENS** + **FIBER** + **CALCIUM**

Makes 4 servings

Brussel sprouts, carrots, and green beans turn sweet and nutty when roasted and topped with a tangy miso dressing. If you've never cooked or eaten anything with nutritional yeast, you're in for a treat. You'll quickly understand why it has earned the nickname "flavor flakes."

---

16 medium Brussels sprouts, halved

1 large carrot, cut into small matchsticks (2 to 3 inches/5 to 7.5 cm long and ¼ inch/6 mm thick)

3½ ounces (100 g) green beans, trimmed and cut into thirds

2 teaspoons extra virgin olive oil

Fine sea salt and black pepper

6 tablespoons (90 ml) warm water

¼ cup (60 g) tahini

6 tablespoons (55 g) nutritional yeast

1 tablespoon white miso paste

1 tablespoon freshly squeezed lemon juice

1 tablespoon minced fresh ginger

---

1 Preheat the oven to 400°F (200°C).

2 Evenly spread the Brussels sprouts, carrot, and green beans on a baking sheet. Drizzle with the oil and season with a pinch each of salt and black pepper. Roast the vegetables for 15 to 18 minutes, until they are easily pierced with a fork but aren't too soft.

3 While the vegetables roast, prepare the dressing by combining the water, tahini, nutritional yeast, miso paste, lemon juice, and ginger in a blender or food processor. Blend until well combined, scraping down the sides as needed.

4 Once the vegetables are cooked, transfer them to a shallow serving dish. Drizzle with the dressing and season to taste with salt and black pepper before serving.

Sweets and Snacks

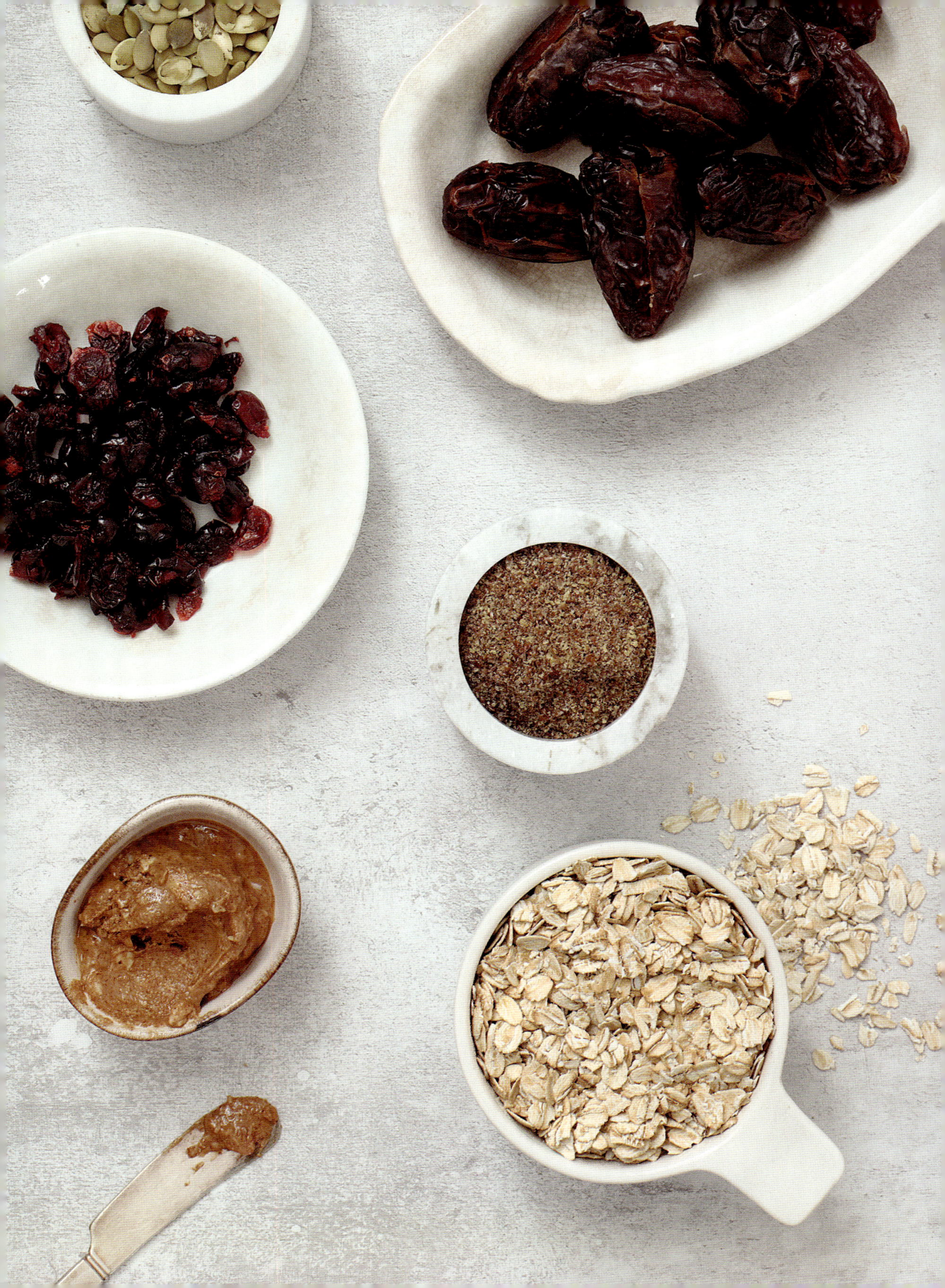

Crunchy Miso Snack and Salad Topper

+ PROTEIN + FIBER

Makes 1½ cups (200 g)

Want to add a quick bit of crunch to your day? Keep a batch of this in your cupboard, and you'll never have to eat a boring salad again. It's not just for salads, though—grab a handful of these flavorful seeds as a quick snack, too.

½ cup (65 g) pumpkin seeds
⅓ cup (30 g) slivered almonds
¼ cup (35 g) raw, unsalted sunflower seeds
¼ cup (35 g) white or black sesame seeds
¼ cup (40 g) whole flax
¼ teaspoon paprika
3 tablespoons tamari
1 teaspoon white or red miso paste
Fine sea salt

---

1 Preheat the oven to 325°F (165°C). Line a baking sheet with parchment paper.

2 Place the pumpkin seeds, almonds, sunflower seeds, sesame seeds, flax, and paprika in a medium bowl. In a separate small bowl, whisk together the tamari and miso paste. Pour the mixture over the seeds and mix until evenly coated.

3 Spread the seed mixture onto the prepared baking sheet and roast for 10 to 12 minutes, until fragrant and lightly golden. Finish with a sprinkle of sea salt, if desired.

4 Allow to cool thoroughly before storing in an airtight container for up to a month.

Rich and Creamy Hummus

Pictured on title page

+ SOY & PHYTOESTROGENS + FIBER + CALCIUM

Makes 6 to 8 servings

Until discovering the secret to homemade hummus, I struggled to find a recipe that came close to the delicious hummus served in my favorite Mediterranean restaurant. The first secret is to overcook the chickpeas (even ones from a can) with baking soda until they're nearly falling apart. The second secret is to use a generous amount of good-quality tahini, which also happens to make this hummus a good source of calcium. Serve as a dip with warm pita bread, or use the hummus as a delicious sandwich spread.

---

1 can (15½ ounces/439 g) chickpeas, rinsed and drained

½ teaspoon baking soda

3 cups (700 ml) water

½ cup (120 g) tahini

¼ cup (60 ml) freshly squeezed lemon juice (about 2 lemons)

1 to 2 cloves garlic, crushed

½ teaspoon fine sea salt, plus more for sprinkling

2 tablespoons ice water, plus more as needed

½ teaspoon ground cumin

1 tablespoon extra virgin olive oil, plus more for drizzling

Pita bread, for serving

---

1 Place the chickpeas and baking soda in a medium saucepan. Pour the 3 cups of water over the chickpeas and bring to a boil over high heat. Cook for 20 minutes, until the chickpeas are very soft. Drain the chickpeas and discard any skins that you can easily remove. Set aside.

2 In a food processor or blender, combine the tahini, lemon juice, garlic, and ½ teaspoon salt and blend until very smooth, scraping down the sides as needed. Add the ice water and blend until the mixture is smooth and velvety. Continue adding ice water, 1 tablespoon at a time, until the mixture is thick but creamy.

continued

3 Add the chickpeas and cumin to the blender. Drizzle in the 1 tablespoon of oil and blend until the mixture is velvety smooth. Add more ice water by the tablespoon if necessary to achieve the desired consistency.

4 Transfer the hummus to a serving dish. Drizzle with oil and sprinkle with sea salt before serving with pita.

5 Store hummus in an airtight container in the refrigerator for up to five days.

White Bean and Pesto Dip

Pictured on title page

+ PROTEIN + FIBER + CALCIUM

Makes 6 to 8 servings

Every year, I ambitiously plant a little vegetable and herb garden. Without fail, I underestimate how difficult it is to grow vegetables and underestimate how easy it is to grow kitchen herbs like basil. When you have a bounty harvest of basil, make this pesto-inspired white bean dip. The garlic, lemon, and basil pair well with the creamy white beans, which also happen to be a good source of iron, along with protein, fiber, and calcium. Serve with pita chips, Miso Flax Crackers (page 212), or your favorite vegetables for dipping.

- 1 can (15½ ounces/439 g) white cannellini beans, rinsed and drained
- ½ cup (20 g) fresh basil leaves
- ¼ cup (60 ml) extra virgin olive oil
- 3 cloves garlic, crushed
- Juice of 1 lemon
- ⅓ cup (35 g) grated Parmesan cheese
- Salt and black pepper
- Pita chips, crackers, or carrot sticks, for serving

---

1 Combine the beans, basil, oil, garlic, and lemon juice in a blender or food processor. Blend until smooth, scraping down the sides as needed. Add the grated parmesan and pulse until just combined.

2 Transfer the dip to a serving dish and serve with pita chips.

3 Store the dip in an airtight container in the refrigerator for up to five days.

Feast on This!

All beans are high in fiber, but white beans—like navy, cannellini, and great northern—are also rich in resistant starch. This type of carbohydrate resists digestion in the small intestine and ferments in the large intestine, producing short-chain fatty acids like butyrate, which can improve gut health, reduce inflammation, and support overall health.

Miso Flax Crackers Pictured on title page

+ SOY & PHYTOESTROGENS + FIBER

Makes 12 to 16 crackers

I'm not usually the kind of person who makes their own crackers, but necessity is the mother of invention, right? After living in the Netherlands for a few years and not being able to find a good seeded cracker to match the ones I used to get in Canada, I set my sights on making my own. These crackers incorporate ground flax and miso paste, providing a well-rounded dose of phytoestrogens.

---

1 cup (120 g) ground flax
¼ cup (40 g) whole flax
2 tablespoons sesame seeds
2 tablespoons pumpkin seeds
1½ teaspoons Italian seasoning
1 teaspoon onion powder
1 teaspoon garlic powder
¼ teaspoon fine sea salt
½ cup (120 ml) lukewarm water
2 teaspoons honey
½ to 1 teaspoon miso paste

---

1 Preheat the oven to 350°F (175°C).

2 Combine the ground flax, whole flax, sesame seeds, pumpkin seeds, Italian seasoning, onion powder, garlic powder, and salt in a medium bowl.

3 In a separate bowl, whisk together the water, honey, and miso paste until completely combined and dissolved.

4 Add the water mixture to the seed mixture and mix well. Let sit for 5 minutes. Transfer the mixture to a piece of parchment paper and work it until it can roughly hold its shape in a ball. This dough will be relatively wet and sticky, so don't compare it to regular dough. Shape the dough into a log about 10 inches (25 cm) in length. Place another piece of parchment paper on top of the dough and use a rolling pin to flatten it to a ⅛-inch (3 mm) thickness.

5 Remove the top layer of parchment paper and transfer the bottom parchment paper and dough to a baking sheet. Score the dough with a knife into the desired cracker shapes and size. Do not try to separate them into pieces before baking.

6 Bake, rotating the pan once, for 20 to 25 minutes, until the crackers are lightly golden with a crispy top. Let cool for 15 minutes before separating and transferring the crackers to a plate. These are deliciously dense and hearty.

7 Once cooled, the crackers can be stored in an airtight container for several days. Reheat for 5 to 8 minutes at 350°F (175°C) if needed to restore their crunchy texture.

FIVE TIPS FOR USING MISO

Miso is a fermented soybean paste that forms the basis of many Japanese dishes. It's also a source of phytoestrogens that can help tame your hot flashes. I like adding it to water when steaming vegetables or making broth to add depth and flavor. Here are a few tips for using miso paste:

1. **Start small and adjust:** Miso can be potent, so start small and gradually add more to taste. This helps avoid overpowering your dish and allows you to fine-tune the flavor balance.
2. **Dissolve before adding:** Dissolve miso in a small amount of warm water or broth before adding it to your dish.
3. **Add miso at the end of cooking:** High heat can diminish miso's delicate flavors, so adding it at the end preserves its taste and nutritional benefits.
4. **Combine with other flavors:** Pair miso with ingredients such as ginger, garlic, soy sauce, and sesame oil. These can enhance miso's umami and create a well-rounded, complex flavor profile in your dishes.
5. **Experiment with different types:** Explore white, yellow, and red miso to discover how each type offers distinct tastes and can be used in various recipes, from light soups and dressings to hearty stews and marinades.

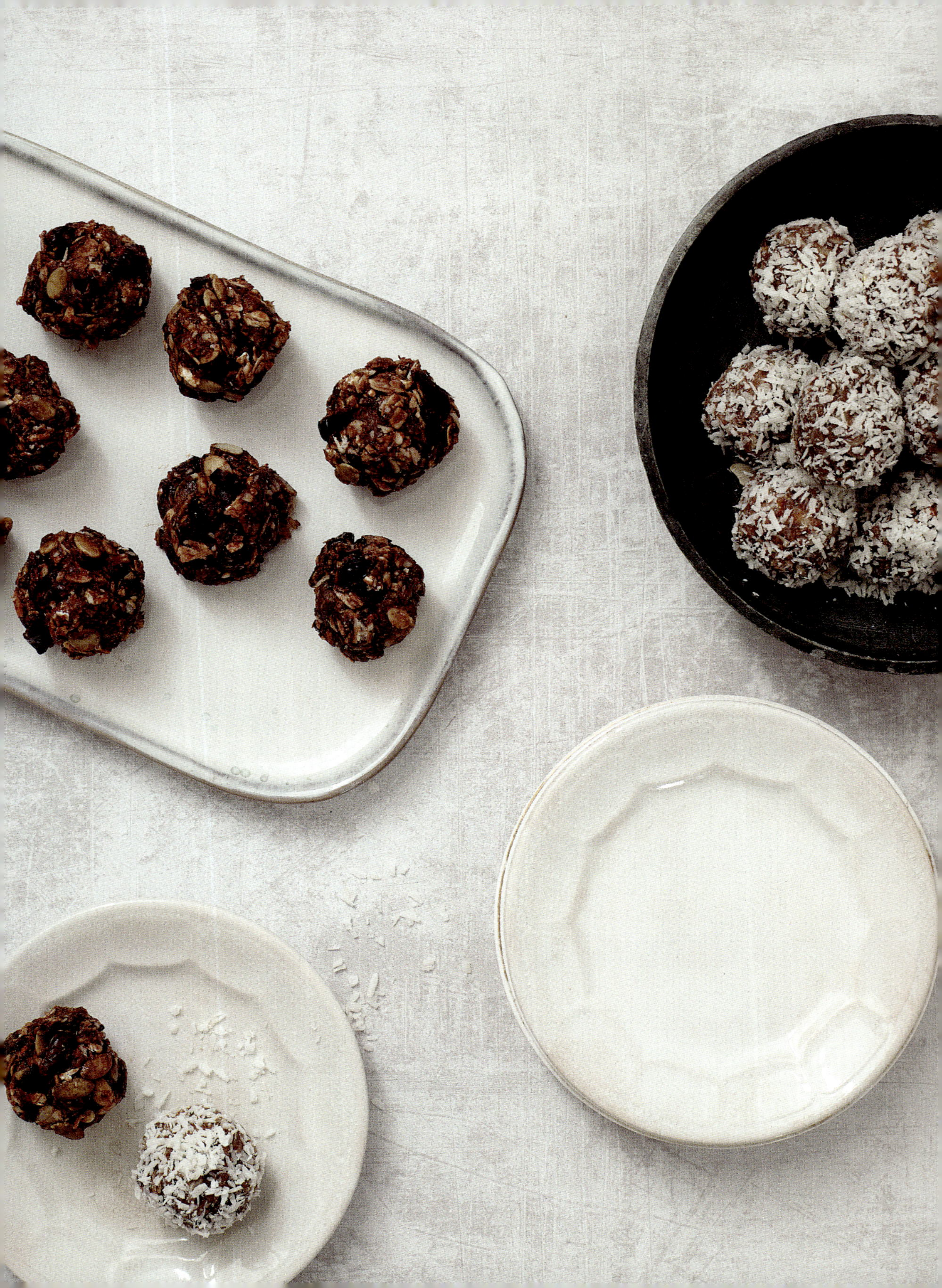

Cranberry Energy Balls

+ SOY & PHYTOESTROGENS + FIBER + OMEGA-3

Makes 12 to 14 balls

When the earthy sweetness of dates meets cranberry and crunch, it's a match made in heaven. The ground flax adds phytoestrgogens and omega-3 fatty acids, while almond butter binds these delightful flavors and textures together. Keep these energy balls—perfect for a post-workout or to-go snack—on hand for when you need a little extra boost.

---

8 to 10 pitted dates, chopped

1 cup (100 g) rolled oats

¼ cup (40 g) dried cranberries, roughly chopped

¼ cup (30 g) pumpkin seeds

¼ cup (30 g) ground flax

2 tablespoons almond butter

---

1 Line a baking sheet with a silicone mat or parchment paper.

2 Using a food processor, pulse the dates until a thick paste forms. Transfer the paste to a medium bowl. Add the oats, cranberries, pumpkin seeds, flax, and almond butter. Mix until well combined. Don't be afraid to use your hands!

3 Roll the mixture into 1-tablespoon balls and place on the prepared baking sheet. You should get 12 to 14 balls. Place the baking sheet in the refrigerator for at least 1 hour before serving.

4 Store in an airtight container in the refrigerator for up to two weeks or freeze for up to two months.

Choco-Flax Balls

+ **SOY & PHYTOESTROGENS** + **FIBER** + **OMEGA-3**

Makes 12 to 14 balls

Nut butter, honey, and cocoa come together in this delightful no-bake snack. Packed with fiber-rich ground flax, oats, and coconut, these bites are perfect for a quick energy boost or as a satisfying dessert. Peppermint extract provides a festive twist, but won't be missed if you'd rather leave it out.

½ cup (145 g) peanut or almond butter

⅓ cup (80 ml) honey

1 cup (100 g) rolled oats

¼ cup (30 g) ground flax

2 tablespoons unsweetened cocoa powder

¼ teaspoon natural peppermint extract or 1 to 2 drops food-grade peppermint essential oil (optional)

Pinch of fine sea salt

2 tablespoons mini chocolate chips, crushed nuts, or candy cane pieces, for mixing (optional)

⅓ cup (30 g) shredded coconut

---

1 Combine the peanut butter and honey in a medium bowl and mix with a fork until smooth. Add the oats, flax, cocoa powder, peppermint extract, if using, and salt. Mix until evenly combined.

2 Fold in the optional ingredients such as chocolate chips, nuts, or candy cane pieces, if using. The mixture should be a bit wet to the touch, which will allow the coconut to stick to the outside.

3 Roll the dough into 1-tablespoon balls and place on a plate. You should have 12 to 14 balls.

4 Pour the coconut onto a small plate or shallow bowl. Gently roll each ball in the shredded coconut. Place on a small plate and refrigerate for at least 30 minutes before serving.

5 Refrigerate in an container up to two weeks or freeze for up to three months.

Blueberry Lemon Flax Muffins

Pictured on page 221

+ **SOY & PHYTOESTROGENS** + **FIBER**

Makes 12 muffins

Sweet and sour is a classic flavor combination, and this recipe brings both to life. Thanks to the staying power of the whole wheat flour and ground flax in the batter, you can count on this muffin to give you a boost any time of day. I love having one with a cup of tea in the afternoon when I'm craving a moment of peace and pleasure.

1½ cups (175 g) whole wheat flour
½ cup (60 g) ground flax
¼ cup (50 g) granulated sugar
1½ teaspoons baking powder
1 teaspoon ground cinnamon
½ teaspoon fine sea salt
1½ cups (350 ml) soy milk
3 tablespoons extra virgin olive oil
2 tablespoons maple syrup or honey
1 large egg
Zest and juice of 1 lemon
2 teaspoons pure vanilla extract
1½ cups (225 g) fresh or frozen blueberries

---

1 Preheat the oven to 375°F (190°C). Grease a muffin tin or line with paper liners.

2 In a large bowl, mix together the flour, flax, sugar, baking powder, cinnamon, and salt. In a separate bowl, whisk together the soy milk, oil, maple syrup, egg, lemon juice and zest, and vanilla.

3 Add the soy milk mixture to the flour mixture. Stir until just combined, then gently fold in the blueberries. Spoon the batter evenly into the prepared muffin tin.

4 Bake for 22 to 25 minutes, or until the tops start to brown and a toothpick inserted in the center of a muffin comes out clean. Cool the muffins in the tin for 5 to 10 minutes before transferring to a cooling rack.

5 Store the muffins in an airtight container on your kitchen counter for up to three days.

Banana Flax Muffins Pictured on page 220

+ SOY & PHYTOESTROGENS + FIBER

Makes 12 muffins

If you love banana bread, then you're going to love this recipe. It's a solution for using up ripe bananas, you only need one bowl to make it, and the muffins can be ready in less than half the time it takes to make banana bread. Add chocolate chips or walnut pieces if you want the muffins to have a little more texture.

½ cup (120 ml) maple syrup or honey
⅓ cup (80 ml) extra virgin olive oil
2 large eggs
2 to 3 medium ripe bananas, mashed
¼ cup (60 ml) soy milk
1¼ cups (145 g) whole wheat flour
⅓ cup (30 g) plus 2 tablespoons rolled oats
¼ cup (30 g) ground flax
1 teaspoon baking soda
1 teaspoon pure vanilla extract
1 teaspoon ground cinnamon
½ teaspoon fine sea salt

---

1 Preheat the oven to 350°F (175°C). Grease a muffin tin or line with paper liners.

2 In a large bowl, whisk together the maple syrup, oil, eggs, bananas, and soy milk. Add the flour, ⅓ cup (30 g) of oats, the flax, baking soda, vanilla, cinnamon, and salt. Mix until just combined.

3 Spoon the batter into the prepared muffin tin so that each cup is about two-thirds full. Sprinkle the tops with the remaining 2 tablespoons of oats. Bake for 20 to 22 minutes, or until a toothpick inserted in the center of a muffin comes out clean. Cool the muffins in the tin for 5 to 10 minutes before transferring to a cooling rack.

4 Store the muffins in an airtight container on your kitchen counter for up to three days.

Food for Thought: What's the Difference Between Whole Flax and Ground Flax?

Whole flax adds a nutty crunch and is an excellent source of fiber, but only ground flax allows us to access the phytoestrogenic lignans that are found in the inner seed. Here are some guidelines for cooking with flax.

WHOLE FLAX

Use: Whole flax can be added to bread, muffins, and other baked goods to add texture and fiber.

Storage: Store whole flax in an airtight container in a cool, dark place for up to a year. For extended freshness, refrigerate or freeze it.

GROUND FLAX (FLAX MEAL)

Use: Ground flax is a source of fiber, lignans (phytoestrogens), and omega-3s. It can be added to smoothies, yogurt, oatmeal, and baked goods.

Substitute for eggs: Mix 1 tablespoon of ground flax with 3 tablespoons of water and let it sit for 5 to 10 minutes to create a flax egg substitute, suitable for baking.

Storage: Ground flax should be stored in an opaque, airtight container in the refrigerator or freezer to maintain freshness for up to three months.

FLAXSEED OIL

Use: Flaxseed oil is best used in cold dishes such as salad dressings and smoothies or drizzled over vegetables. Avoid using flaxseed oil for cooking because it has a low smoke point and can lose its nutritional benefits when heated.

Storage: Flaxseed oil should be stored in the refrigerator in an opaque, airtight container to prevent oxidation. Use it within a few months of opening to ensure freshness.

BAKING WITH FLAX

Incorporating flax: You can replace up to 25 percent of the flour in baked goods with ground flax. This will add protein, fiber, and a slightly nutty flavor to your recipes. The unsaturated fats in flax can tolerate baking temperatures up to 375°F (190°C).

Hydration: Flax can absorb a significant amount of water, so you may need to increase the liquid content of your recipes slightly to maintain the desired consistency.

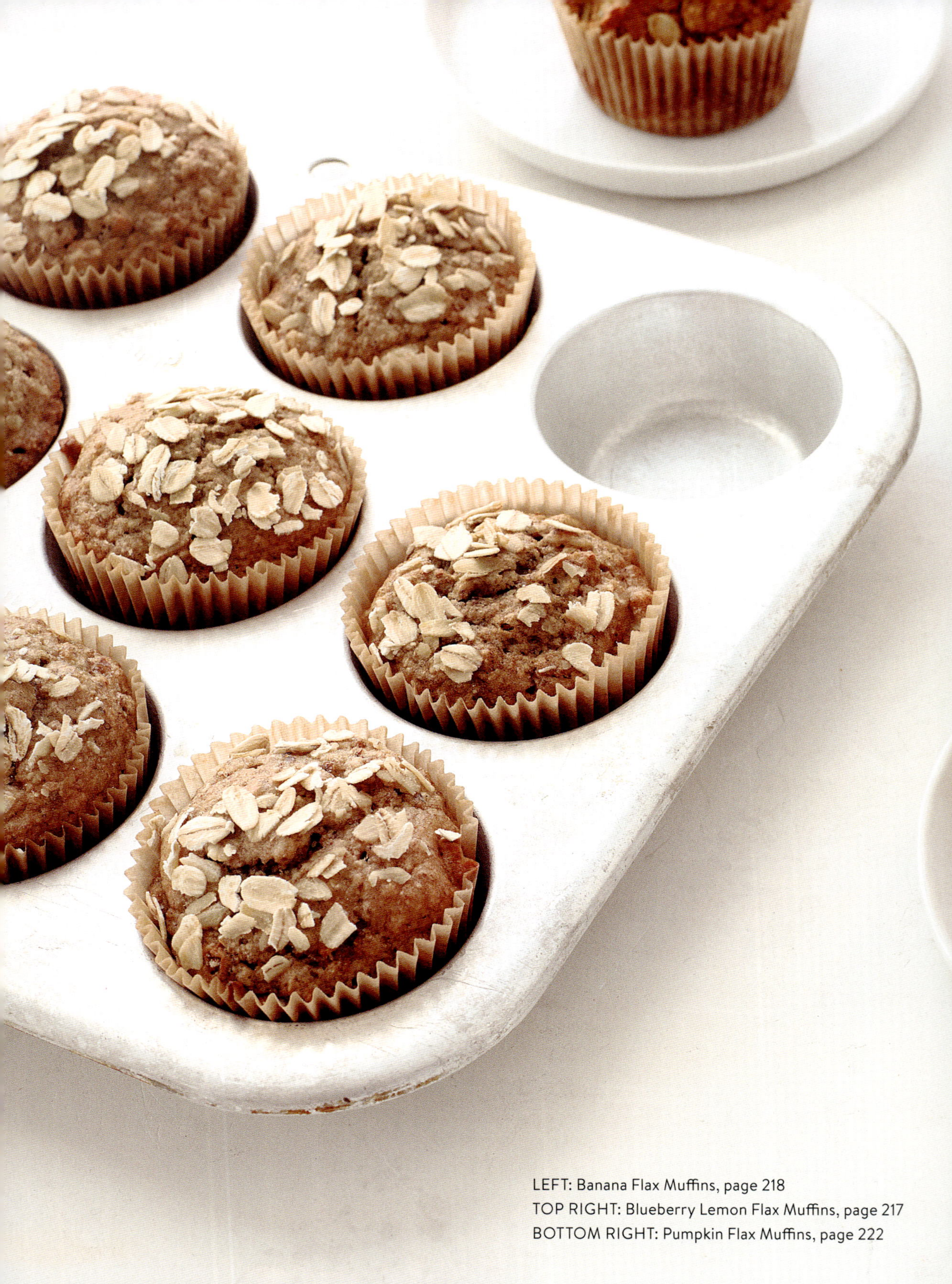

LEFT: Banana Flax Muffins, page 218
TOP RIGHT: Blueberry Lemon Flax Muffins, page 217
BOTTOM RIGHT: Pumpkin Flax Muffins, page 222

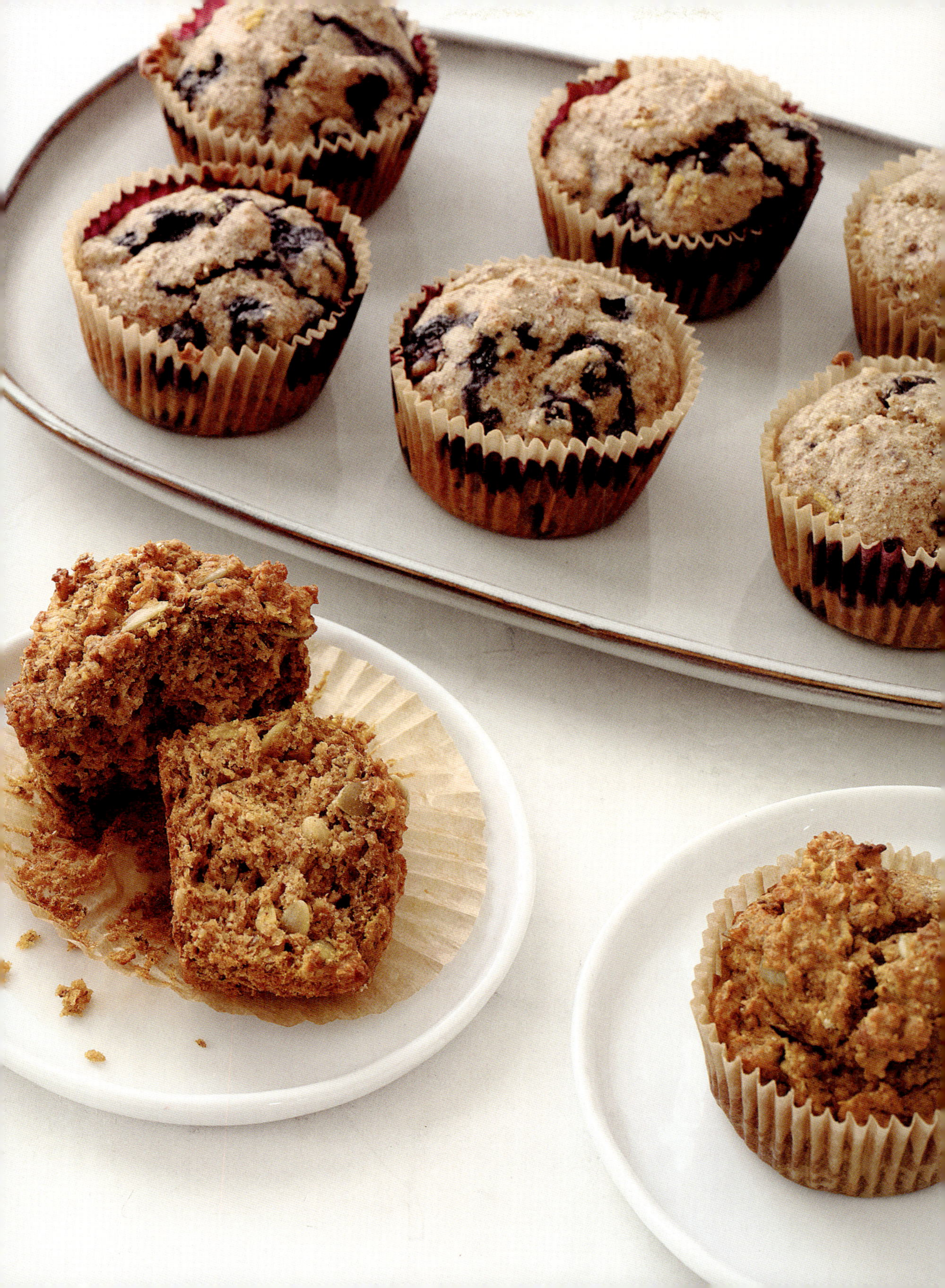

Pumpkin Flax Muffins Pictured on page 221

+ SOY & PHYTOESTROGENS + FIBER

Makes 12 muffins

Everyone needs a go-to muffin recipe that's on repeat. Don't be fooled into thinking this is a seasonal recipe, as canned pumpkin makes this recipe easy to pull together year-round.

½ cup (120 ml) maple syrup or honey

⅓ cup (80 ml) extra virgin olive oil

2 large eggs

1 cup (245 g) pumpkin puree

¼ cup (60 ml) soy milk

1 teaspoon baking soda

1 teaspoon pure vanilla extract

¾ teaspoon ground cinnamon (see note)

¾ teaspoon ground ginger (see note)

½ teaspoon baking powder

½ teaspoon fine sea salt

¼ teaspoon ground nutmeg (see note)

¼ teaspoon ground allspice or cloves (see note)

1¼ cups (145 g) whole wheat flour

⅓ cup (30 g) rolled oats

⅓ cup (45 g) pumpkin seeds

¼ cup (30 g) ground flax

⅓ cup (60 g) chocolate chips or chopped nuts (optional)

1 Preheat the oven to 350°F (175°C). Grease a muffin tin or line with paper liners.

2 In a large bowl, whisk together the maple syrup and oil. Add the eggs, pumpkin puree, soy milk, baking soda, vanilla, cinnamon, ginger, baking powder, salt, nutmeg, and allspice. Mix in the flour, oats, pumpkin seeds, and flax until just combined. Add the chocolate chips, if using.

3 Spoon the batter evenly into the prepared muffin tin and bake for 22 to 25 minutes, until a toothpick inserted in the center of a muffin comes out clean. Cool the muffins in the tin for 5 to 10 minutes before transferring to a cooling rack.

4 Store the muffins in an airtight container for up to three days.

Note: You can use 2 teaspoons of pumpkin pie spice instead of cinnamon, ginger, nutmeg, and allspice.

Tofu Pudding

+ SOY & PHYTOESTROGENS + FIBER + CALCIUM

Makes 4 to 6 servings

Silken tofu is ideal for making puddings, thanks to its rich and creamy texture. Much like other types of tofu, it's happy to take on the taste of whatever it's being paired with. In this recipe, the dark chocolate, vanilla, and salt bring the pudding to life.

---

6 ounces (170 g) dark 70% chocolate, roughly chopped

1 package (12 ounces/340 g) silken tofu, drained

3 tablespoons cocoa powder

2 tablespoons maple syrup

1 tablespoon brown sugar

1 teaspoon pure vanilla extract

Coarse sea salt

---

1 Melt the chocolate either in a microwave or on the stovetop. For the microwave, put the chocolate in a microwave-safe bowl and melt in 30-second bursts, stirring in between to prevent burning. For the stovetop, place 2 inches (5 cm) of water in a saucepan and place a heatproof bowl with the chocolate over the top, making sure the water does not reach the bottom of the bowl. Bring the water to a boil, then reduce the heat so the water is simmering. Stir until the chocolate is melted. Once melted, set aside.

2 Combine the tofu, cocoa powder, maple syrup, brown sugar, and vanilla in a food processor or blender and blend until smooth, scraping down the sides as needed. Pour in the melted chocolate and blend again until well combined.

3 Spoon the pudding into ramekins or small bowls and refrigerate for at least 30 minutes. Sprinkle with sea salt before serving.

4 To keep the pudding for later, put it in an airtight container (or spoon into ramekins and cover with plastic wrap) and store in the refrigerator for up to five days.

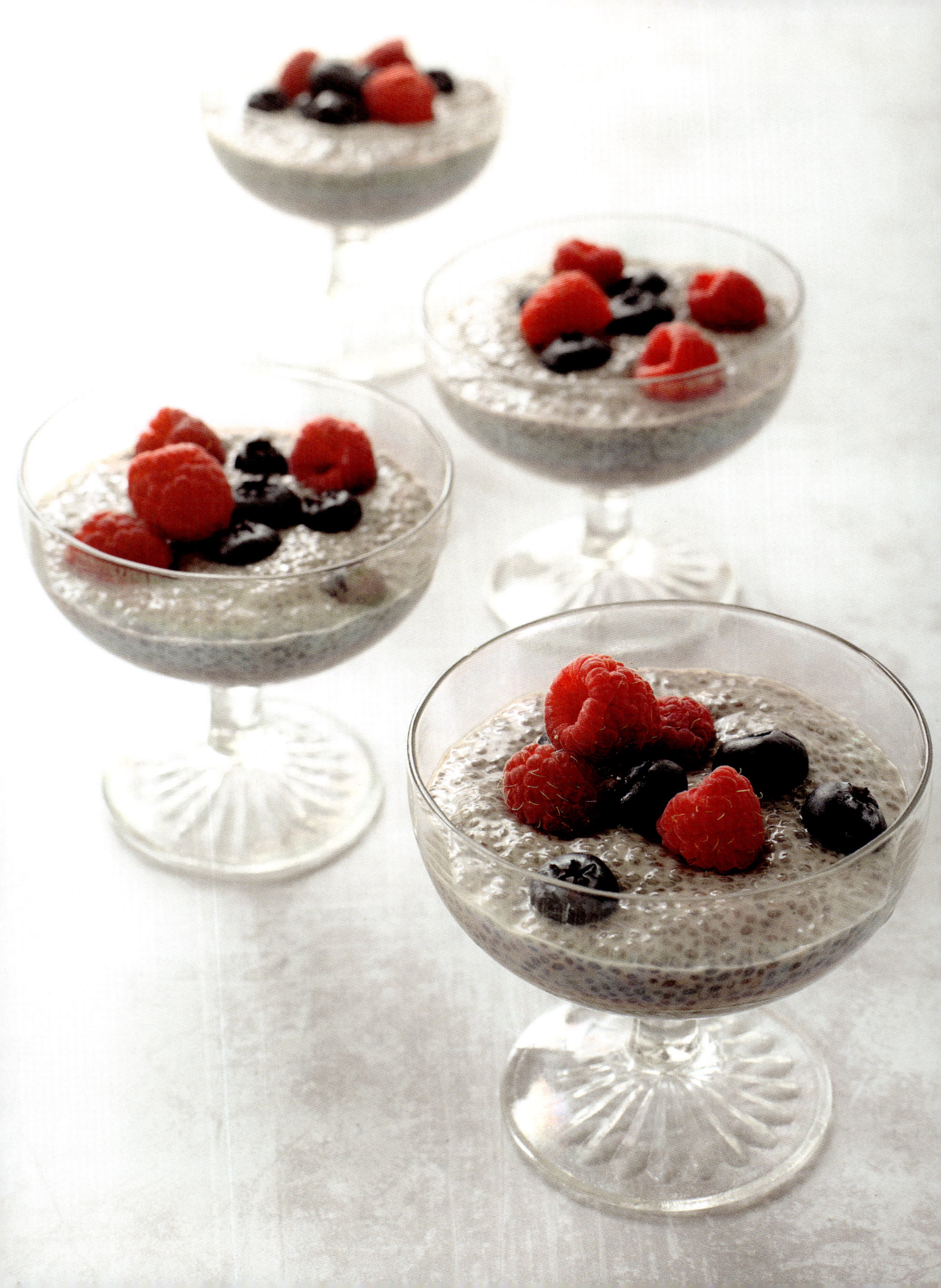

Chia Seed Pudding

+ **SOY & PHYTOESTROGENS** + **PROTEIN** + **FIBER** + **CALCIUM** + **OMEGA-3**

Makes 2 to 4 servings

Chia pudding makes a nourishing breakfast that includes all the key ingredients you need in midlife. You can make the pudding ahead, and it'll be ready for your morning meal, but you can also have it as a midday snack or dessert. I usually eat chia pudding on its own, but adding a spoonful or two to your morning oatmeal or yogurt is another way to enjoy it.

---

2 cups (475 ml) soy milk
½ cup (85 g) black chia seeds (see note)
1 to 2 tablespoons maple syrup (depending on your desired sweetness)
1 teaspoon pure vanilla extract
1 teaspoon unsweetened cocoa powder
Berries of choice, for serving

---

1 Place the soy milk, chia seeds, maple syrup, vanilla, and cocoa powder in a medium bowl and stir well. Cover and refrigerate for at least 4 hours.

2 In the morning or when ready to eat, uncover and thoroughly mix with a spoon as the chia seeds often sink to the bottom. Top with berries and serve.

3 Put the pudding in an airtight container (without the berries) and store it in the refrigerator for up to five days.

Note: Some people find that chia seeds have a tendency to get stuck in their teeth. This can easily be remedied by pulsing the seeds in an immersion blender before using them.

Creamy Rice Pudding
with Ginger and Vanilla

+ **SOY & PHYTOESTROGENS** + **CALCIUM**

Makes 4 to 6 servings

Rice pudding was one of my dad's favorite desserts, and I remember his excitement the first time I prepared it from scratch. Comforting and cozy, rice pudding made with soy milk means it's a delicious way to add a dose of soy and phytoestrogens to the dish. Fresh ginger adds another layer of warmth to this nourishing dessert.

½ cup (90 g) uncooked long-grain rice

1 cup (240 ml) water

3 cups (700 ml) soy milk

¼ cup (55 g) packed brown sugar

1 cinnamon stick

2 teaspoons pure vanilla extract

1 piece (1½ inches/4 cm) fresh ginger, grated

¼ cup (40 g) raisins (optional)

Pinch of fine sea salt

---

1 In a colander placed in the sink, wash and drain the rice until the water runs clear. Place the rice and water in a medium saucepan and bring to a boil over high heat. Cover, reduce the heat to low, and simmer for 10 minutes, until rice has started to soften, taking care not to let all the water evaporate from the rice.

2 Add the soy milk, brown sugar, cinnamon stick, vanilla, half of the ginger, and raisins, if using, to the pan. Stir well and simmer on low, uncovered and stirring occasionally, for 20 to 25 minutes, until the pudding looks like a thick and creamy porridge. Remove from the heat and mix in the remaining ginger and the salt. Remove the cinnamon stick and stir well.

3 Serve warm in parfait glasses or dessert bowls.

4 To keep for later, let the pudding cool, then transfer to an airtight container and store it in the refrigerator for up to three days.

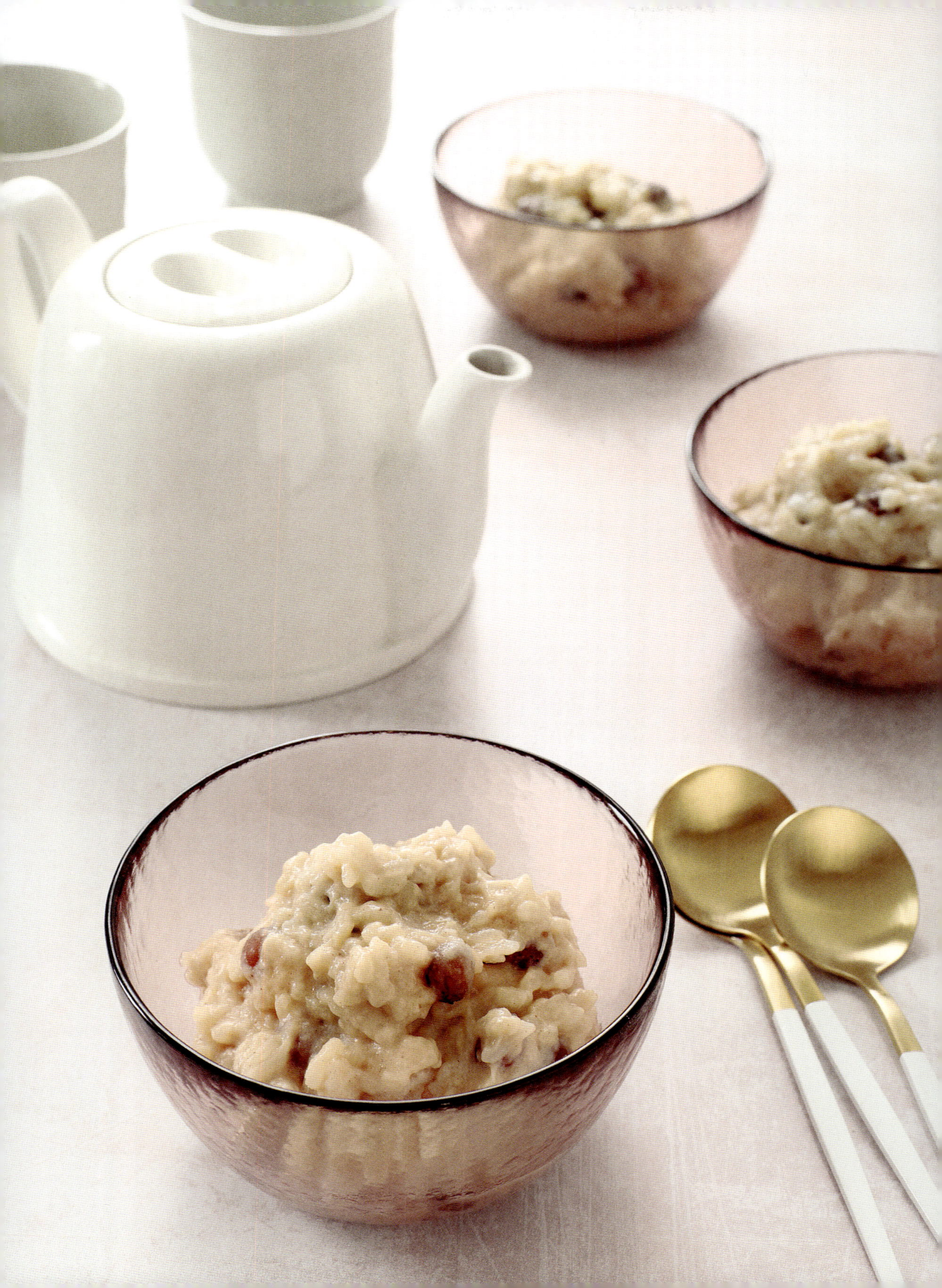

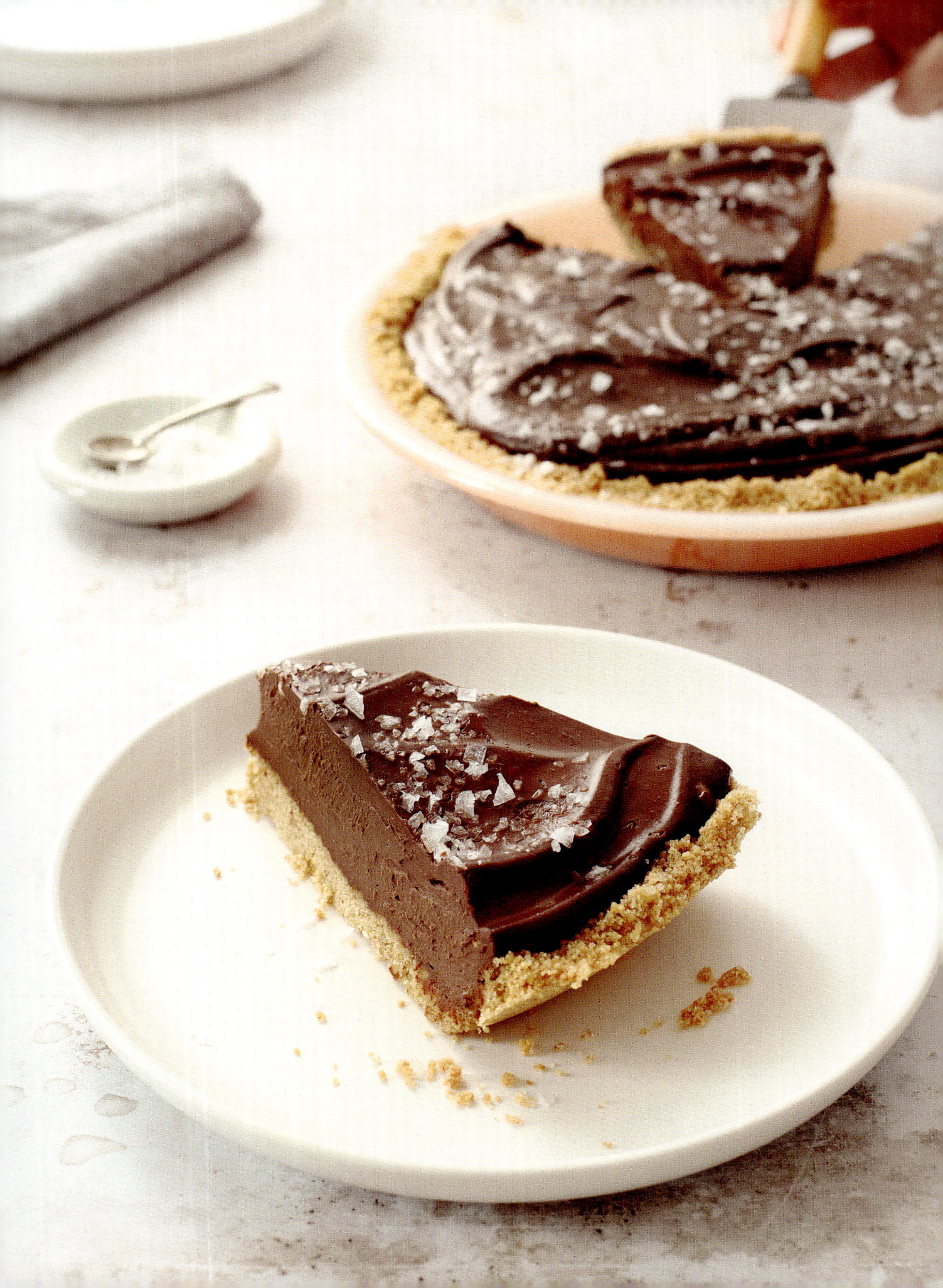

No-Bake Peanut Butter Chocolate Tofu Pie

+ SOY & PHYTOESTROGENS + PROTEIN + FIBER + OMEGA 3

Makes 8 servings

Is there any better combination than peanut butter and chocolate? They make a great no-bake dessert in this refrigerator pie. Silken tofu's rich and creamy texture puts this dessert high on the list of must-have recipes. It comes together quickly with a premade graham cracker crust, but you can always make your own if you prefer.

1 package (12 ounces/340 g) silken tofu, drained

½ cup (120 ml) soy milk

½ cup (145 g) natural peanut butter

¼ cup (20 g) unsweetened cocoa powder

12 ounces (340 g) semisweet (60%) chocolate

1 prepared graham cracker crust

Pinch of flaky sea salt

1 In a blender, combine the tofu, soy milk, peanut butter, and cocoa powder and pulse until smooth. Scrape down the sides of the blender as needed.

2 Melt the chocolate either in a microwave or on the stovetop. For the microwave, put the chocolate in a microwave-safe bowl and melt in 30-second bursts, stirring in between to prevent burning. For the stovetop, place 2 inches (5 cm) of water in a small saucepan and place a heatproof bowl with the chocolate over the top, making sure the bottom of the bowl does not touch the water. Bring the water to a boil, then reduce the heat so the water is simmering. Stir until the chocolate is melted.

3 Working in batches, slowly add the melted chocolate to the tofu mixture and blend until smooth.

4 Use a spatula to transfer the filling to the prepared crust. Sprinkle the sea salt on top, then chill for at least 6 hours. Remove from the refrigerator when you're ready to slice and serve.

5 Leftovers will keep for three days, covered, in the refrigerator.

Cooling and Comforting Drinks

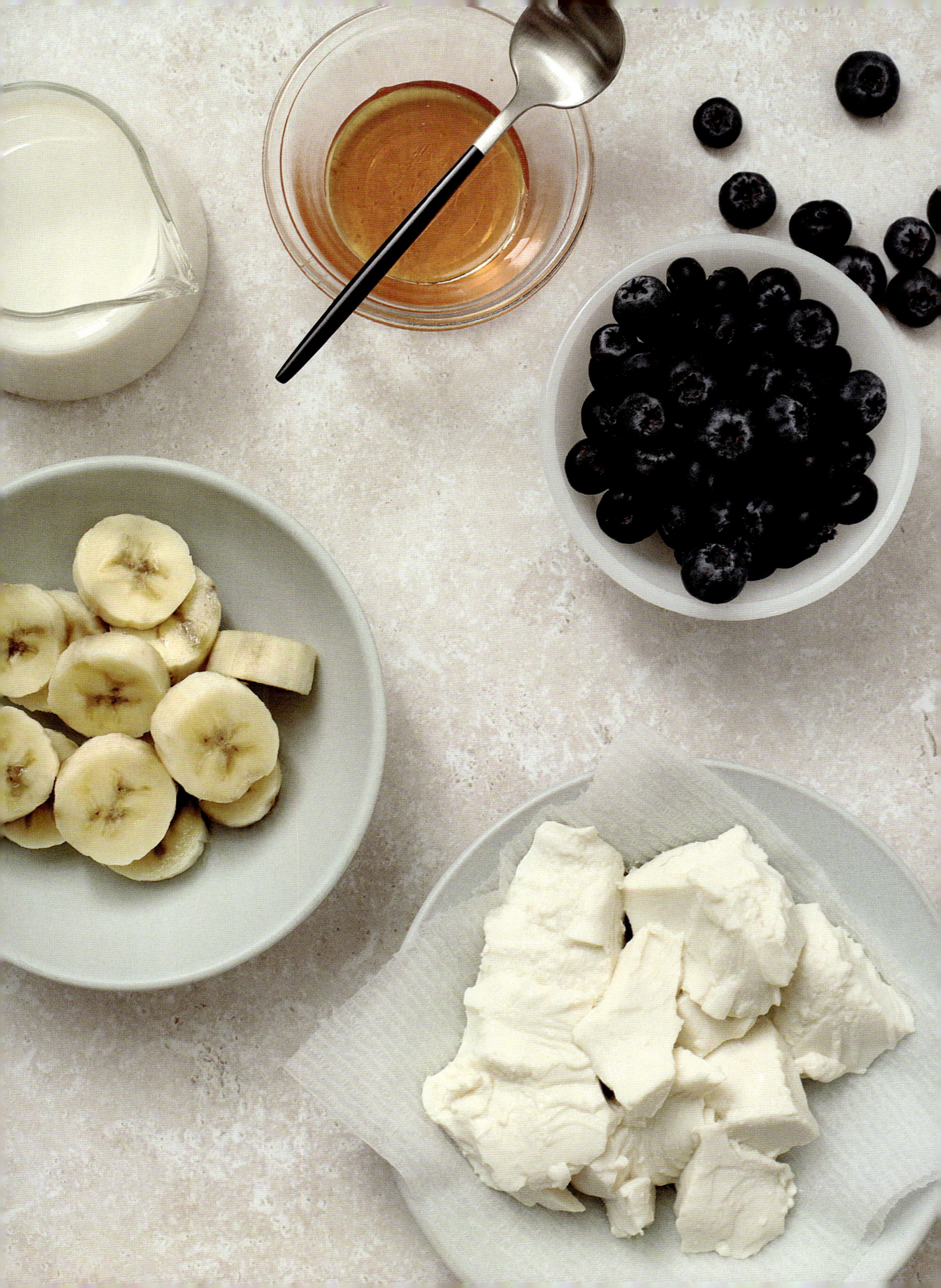

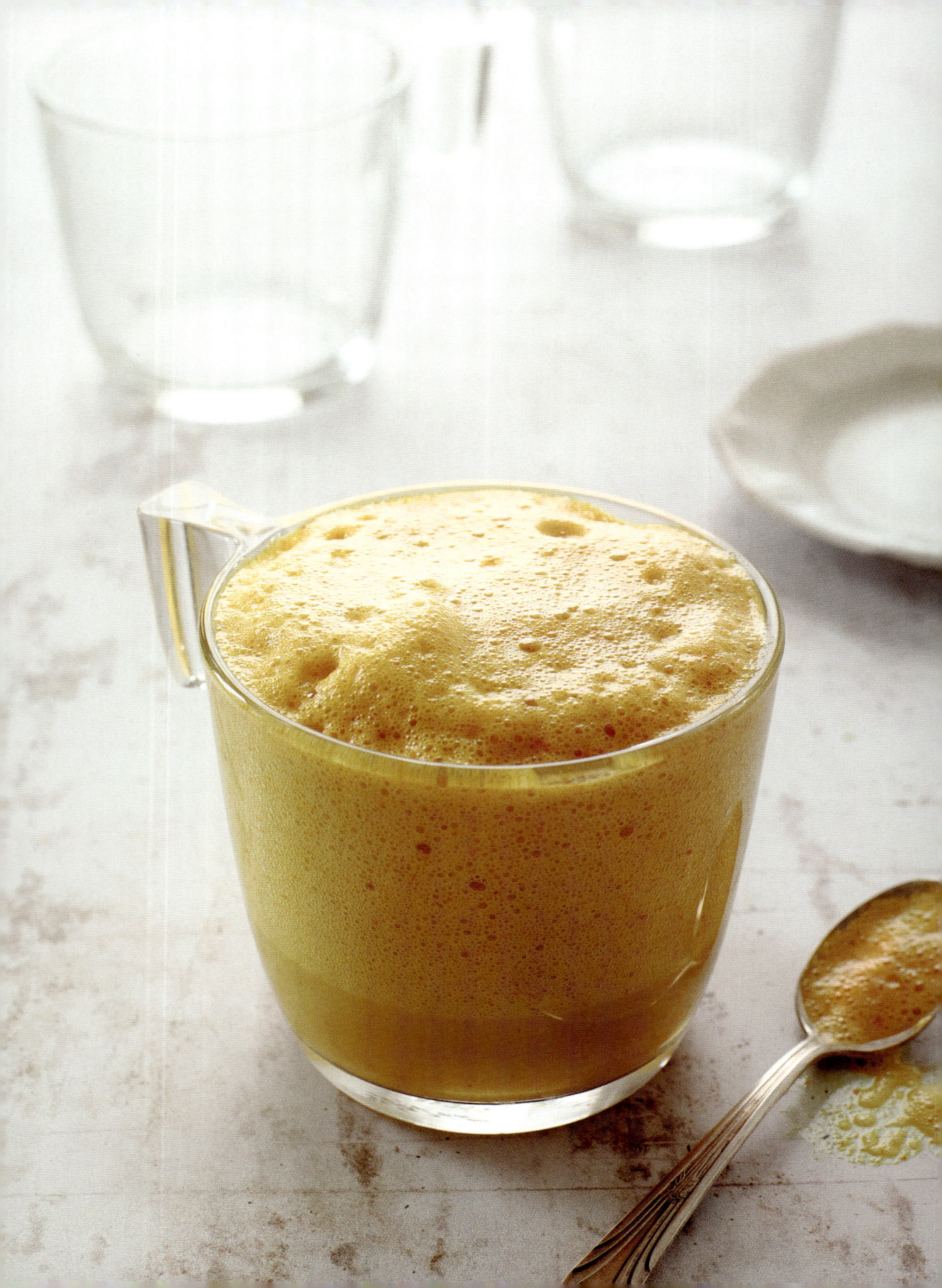

Golden Soy Latte

+ **SOY & PHYTOESTROGENS** + **PROTEIN** + **CALCIUM**

Makes 1 serving

This golden latte, a spin on golden milk, is comfort in a cup and draws on the warming spices of turmeric and ginger. To make the drink more filling and satisfying, add a scoop of vanilla protein powder.

---

1 cup (240 ml) soy milk

1 scoop (30 g) of vanilla protein powder (optional)

1 to 2 teaspoons maple syrup or honey (depending on how sweet you want the drink)

1½ teaspoons ground turmeric

½ teaspoon ground ginger

Pinch of black pepper

---

1 Pour the soy milk into a small saucepan and place over low heat. If using the protein powder, whisk it into the soy milk until no lumps are visible.

2 Add the maple syrup, turmeric, ginger, and black pepper and stir. Warm for 3 to 5 minutes, stirring constantly, being careful not to let it burn.

3 When slightly steaming, remove from the heat and serve. If you have a milk frother, you can use it to whip some air into your latte before serving.

Feast on This!

Golden milk made with turmeric is a popular drink from India, where it's enjoyed as a home remedy for a variety of ailments. One study compared the properties of different golden milk drinks when made with either cow milk, part-skimmed cow milk, or soy milk, at various concentrations and temperatures. Of the various milks, they found that the one made with soy milk had the highest concentration of antioxidant activity.[1]

Blueberry Banana Tofu Smoothie

+ SOY & PHYTOESTROGENS + PROTEIN + CALCIUM + OMEGA-3

Makes 2 to 4 servings

My relationship with smoothies has evolved over the years. I once used them to cram in as much nutrition as I possibly could into a single meal (usually breakfast). I now welcome them as a convenient and satisfying way to make menopause nutrition feel easy and help keep my hot flashes at bay. Silken tofu's high water content is ideal for blending and creates a rich and creamy base for this fresh smoothie. Use the ice cubes if you like a thicker, colder smoothie.

---

1 cup (240 ml) soy milk

6 ounces (170 g) silken tofu, drained

1 medium ripe banana, sliced

1 cup (150 g) fresh or frozen blueberries

1 tablespoon honey

2 to 3 ice cubes (optional)

---

1 Combine the soy milk, tofu, and banana in a blender and blend for 30 seconds. Add half of the blueberries. Blend again until combined.

2 Add the remaining blueberries, the honey, and ice cubes, if using, and continue blending until smooth.

3 This smoothie is best enjoyed right away.

4 If you haven't used the ice, it can keep in an airtight container in the refrigerator for up to one day.

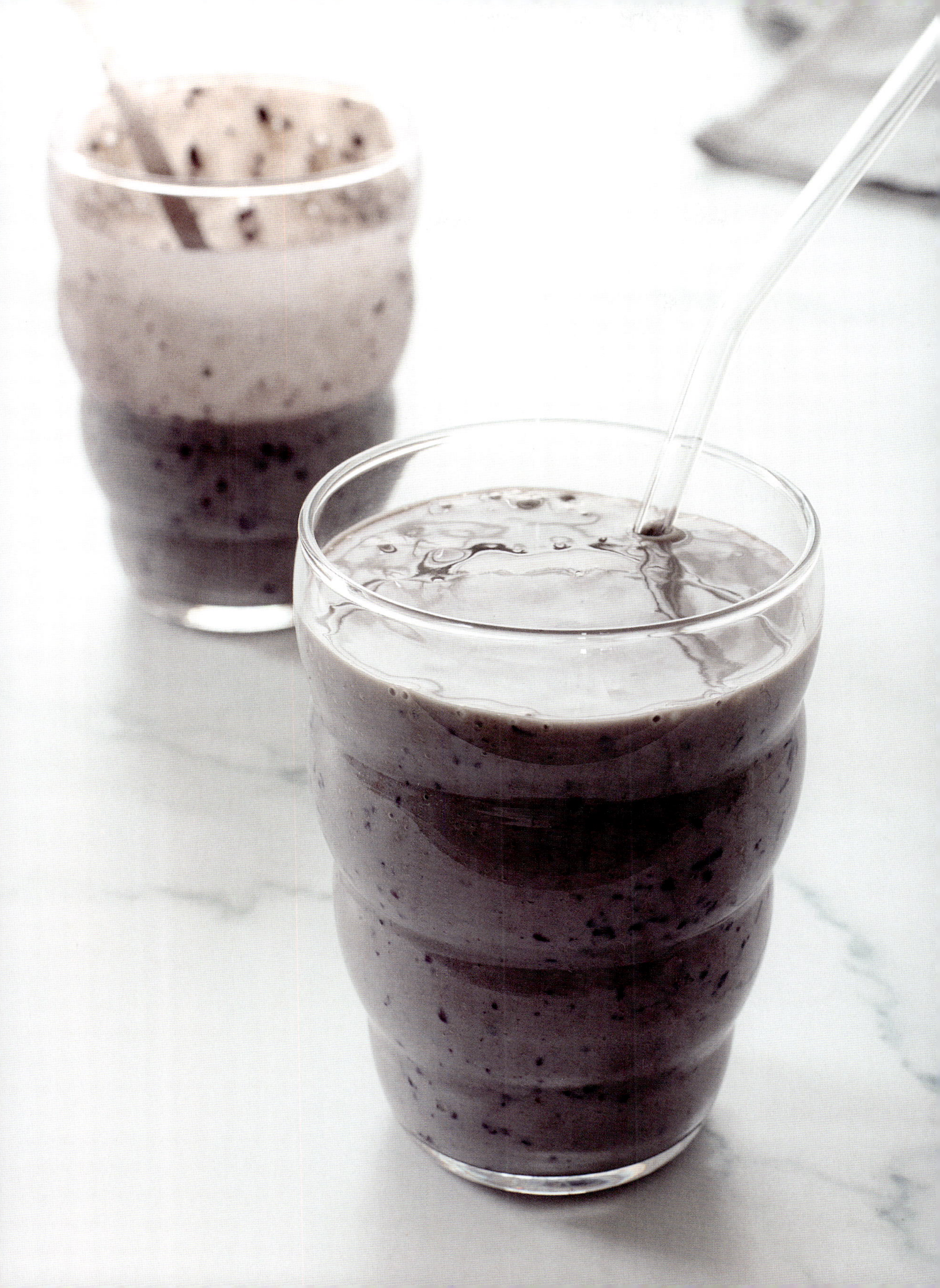

Chocolate and Chill Smoothie

+ **SOY & PHYTOESTROGENS** + **PROTEIN** + **FIBER** + **CALCIUM** + **OMEGA-3**

Makes 1 serving

This smoothie is perfect for those moments when you're craving something cool, refreshing, and satisfying. The mix of chocolate and peppermint flavors hits the spot, while the other ingredients do the heavy lifting of making the drink both balanced and packed with nutrition. Add crushed ice for an extra cooling effect—when a hot flash strikes or simply on a hot day.

---

1 cup (240 ml) unsweetened soy milk

1 medium ripe banana, sliced

1 scoop chocolate-flavored protein powder

1 large handful baby spinach

1 tablespoon hemp hearts

2 teaspoons pure maple syrup

1 teaspoon cocoa powder

¼ to ½ teaspoon peppermint extract (adjust to your taste preference)

Crushed ice (optional)

---

1 Combine the soy milk, banana, protein powder, spinach, hemp hearts, maple syrup, cocoa powder, peppermint extract, and ice, if using, in a blender and blend on high for 30 to 60 seconds until smooth and no lumps remain.

2 This smoothie is best enjoyed right away.

3 If you haven't used the ice, it will keep in an airtight container in the refrigerator for up to one day.

Cranberry Mocktail Festive Spritzer

Pictured on page 240

Makes 1 serving

I love the color of this vibrant cranberry mocktail that packs the perfect punch of sweet and sour. Despite its festive name and appearance, it's one you can enjoy all year long, especially if you want to forgo traditional cocktails.

¼ cup (60 ml) of 100% cranberry juice

2 tablespoons Simple Honey Syrup (recipe follows)

1 tablespoon freshly squeezed lemon or lime juice

Ice

Club soda, for topping

Sprig of rosemary and frozen cranberries, for garnish

---

1 In a cocktail shaker, combine the cranberry juice, honey syrup, and lemon juice. Add ice to the shaker and shake vigorously for 10 to 15 seconds, until well mixed and chilled.

2 Strain into a highball glass with ice and top with club soda. Add a sprig of rosemary and a few frozen cranberries on top for a festive garnish. Enjoy.

continued

Simple Honey Syrup

Makes 1 cup (240 ml)

A simple honey syrup can be made ahead to keep in your fridge. Use it as the base for spritzer mocktails (page 237 and opposite).

½ cup (120 ml) water

½ cup (120 ml) honey

1 Combine the water and honey in a small saucepan over medium heat. Bring to a boil, stirring constantly, until the honey is completely dissolved in the water. Remove from the heat and let cool completely.

2 Refrigerate the simple syrup in an airtight container for up to one month.

Citrus and Honey Summer Spritzer Pictured on page 241

Makes 1 serving

Many women discover that their tolerance for alcohol changes in midlife, and even a single glass of wine can wreak havoc on both sleep and body temperature. A beautifully crafted mocktail, however, offers all the flavor and sophistication without the side effects. It's a mindful choice that allows you to savor an evening, stay present, and wake up feeling refreshed the next day. This warm-weather mocktail combines the bright, tangy flavors of grapefruit and lime, sweetened with a touch of homemade simple honey syrup. Topped with fizzy club soda, it's a light and invigorating drink that's perfect for any time of day.

¼ cup (60 ml) fresh grapefruit juice

2 tablespoons Simple Honey Syrup (see opposite)

2 tablespoons freshly squeezed lime juice

Ice

Club soda, for topping

Twist of grapefruit peel, for garnish

---

1 In a cocktail shaker, combine the grapefruit juice, honey syrup, and lime juice. Fill the shaker with ice and shake vigorously for 10 to 15 seconds, until well mixed and chilled.

2 Strain into a highball glass with ice and top with club soda. Add a twist of grapefruit peel on top for garnish. Serve immediately and enjoy.

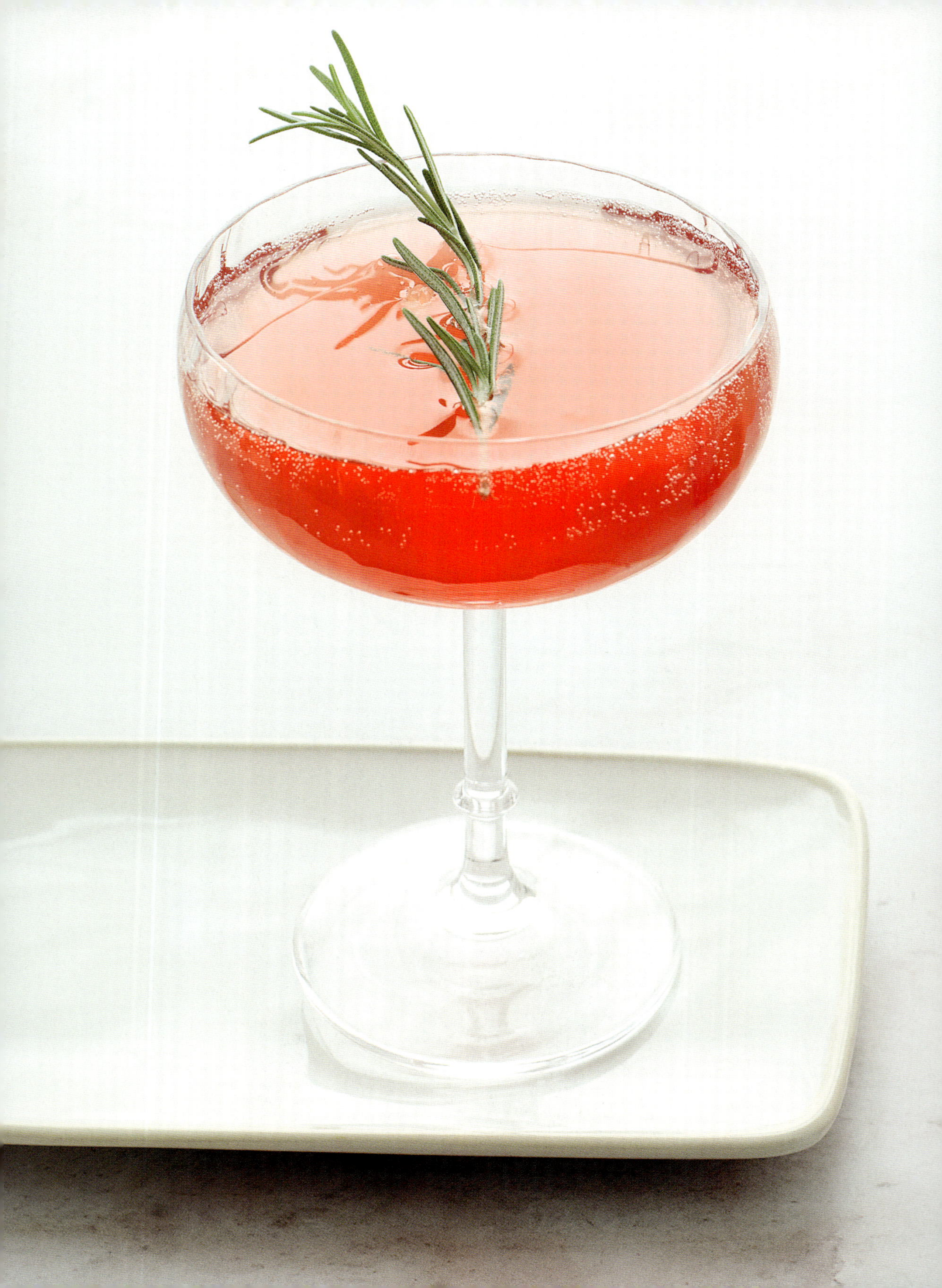

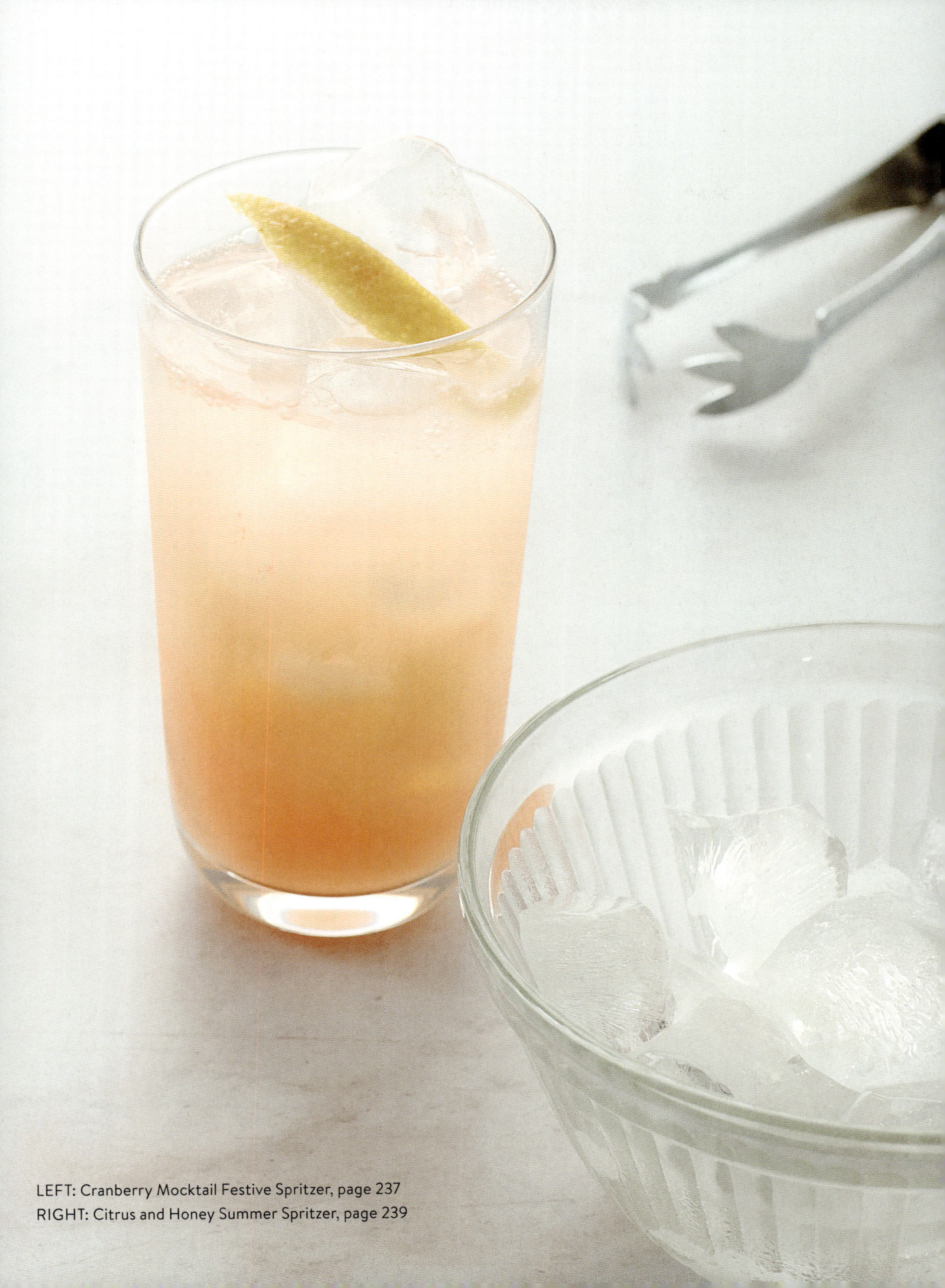
LEFT: Cranberry Mocktail Festive Spritzer, page 237
RIGHT: Citrus and Honey Summer Spritzer, page 239

Help Me Quickly Hot Flash Meal Plan!

Here's a week of phytoestrogen- and isoflavone-rich meal ideas to help bring down the temperature of your hot flashes. Keep in mind that it may take a few weeks of eating soy and phytoestrogen-rich foods before you notice a consistent cooling effect.

	SUNDAY	MONDAY	TUESDAY
BREAKFAST	Tofu Scramble	Key Lime Overnight Oats	Breakfast burrito with leftover Tofu Scramble
LUNCH	Savory Sweet Potato Egg Bites	Tuna Salad with Cranberry	Smashed Chickpea Salad in a whole wheat wrap
DINNER	Saucy Slow-Cooked Tikka Masala	Tofu Broccoli Salad with Kimchi Miso Dressing served with rice	Sweet Potato Salmon Cakes served with salad or fries
SNACK	Banana Flax Muffin	Chocolate and Chill Smoothie	Pumpkin Flax Muffin

Includes 7 to 10 servings of soy and phytoestrogen-rich meals, providing 25 to 50 mg of isoflavones.

Other quick and easy ways to include isoflavones:

Soy milk (1 cup/240 ml) = 25 mg

Soy nuts (⅓ cup/30 g) = 45 mg

Shelled edamame (½ cup/80 g) = 16 mg

WEDNESDAY	THURSDAY	FRIDAY	SATURDAY
Pumpkin Smoothie Bowl	Tiramisu Overnight Oats	Blueberry Banana Tofu Smoothie	Whipped Cottage Cheese Parfait
Cilantro Black Bean Salad and tortilla chips	Spinach and Mozzarella Pita Pizza	Leftover Spicy Black Bean Burgers added to a salad or grain bowl	PB&J sandwich made with Very Berry Chia Jam on whole grain bread
Marinated Tofu and Soba Noodles with Bok Choy	Spicy Black Bean Burgers	Potato Chickpea Curry	Sheet-Pan Pistachio-Crusted Fish and Roasted Potatoes
Tofu Pudding	Chia Seed Pudding	Choco-Flax Balls	Miso Flax Crackers with Rich and Creamy Hummus

ENDNOTES

PREFACE

1 K. Hill, "The Demography of Menopause," *Maturitas* 23, no. 2 (March 1996): 113–127, https://doi.org/10.1016/0378-5122(95)00968-x.

2 G. F. H. McLeod, L. Cleland, J. Welch, J. K. Spittlehouse, A. Fenton, J. M. Boden, et al., "Menopause Status and Climacteric Symptoms in a Birth Cohort of Mid-Life New Zealand Women," *Climacteric* 25, no. 3 (June 2022): 271–277, https://doi.org/10.1080/13697137.2021.1948005.

3 "Menopause and Bone Loss," Endocrine Society, updated January 24, 2022, https://www.endocrine.org/patient-engagement/endocrine-library/menopause-and-bone-loss.

INTRODUCTION

1 S. M. Hofmeier, C. D. Runfola, M. Sala, D. A. Gagne, K. A. Brownley, and C. M. Bulik, "Body Image, Aging, and Identity in Women Over 50: The Gender and Body Image (Gabi) Study," *J Women Aging* 29, no. 1 (January/February 2017): 3–14, https://doi.org/10.1080/08952841.2015.1065140.

2 K. E. Campbell, L. Dennerstein, S. Finch, and C. E. Szoeke, "Impact of Menopausal Status on Negative Mood and Depressive Symptoms in a Longitudinal Sample Spanning 20 Years," *Menopause* 24, no. 5 (May 2017): 490–496, https://doi.org/10.1097/GME.0000000000000805.

3 S. Vestergaard, M. Thinggaard, B. Jeune, J. W. Vaupel, M. McGue, and K. Christensen, "Physical and Mental Decline and Yet Rather Happy? A Study of Danes Aged 45 and Older," *Aging Mental Health* 19, no. 5 (2015): 400–408, https://doi.org/10.1080/13607863.2014.944089.

4 "By the Numbers," *Annual Report*, National Women's Business Council, 2023, https://www.nwbc.gov/annual-reports/2023/BytheNumbers.html.

5 H. G. Burger, A. H. MacLennan, K. E. Huang, and C. Castelo-Branco, "Evidence-Based Assessment of the Impact of the WHI on Women's Health," *Climacteric* 15, no. 3 (June 2012): 281–287, https://doi.org/10.3109/13697137.2012.655564.

6 "2022 Food and Health Survey," Food Insight, May 18, 2022, https://foodinsight.org/2022-food-and-health-survey.

7 OECD and the Food and Agriculture Organization of the United States, "Protein Intake Per Capita on Least Developed, Other Developing and Developed Countries," in *OECD-FAO Agricultural Outlook 2015*, https://doi.org/10.1787/agr_outlook-2015-graph8-en.

8 Common Sense Media, "New Report by Common Sense Media Reveals Kids' Body Image Develops as Early as Five and Media and Parents Play Pivotal Role," news release, January 21, 2015, https://www.commonsensemedia.org/press -releases/new-report-by-common-sense-media -reveals-kids-body-image-develops-as-early-as -five-and-media-and-parents.

9 N. Van Dyke and E. J. Drinkwater, "Relationships Between Intuitive Eating and Health Indicators: Literature Review," *Public Health Nutrition* 17, no. 8 (August 2014): 1757–1766, https://doi.org/10.1017/S1368980013002139.

10 M. J. Christoph, V. M. Hazzard, E. Järvelä-Reijonen, L. Hooper, N. Larson, and D. Neumark-Sztainer, "Intuitive Eating Is Associated with Higher Fruit and Vegetable Intake Among Adults," *Journal of Nutrition Education and Behavior* 53, no. 3 (March 2021): 240–245, https://doi.org/10.1016/j.jneb.2020.11.015.

11 J. Linardon, T. L. Tylka, and M. Fuller-Tyszkiewicz, "Intuitive Eating and Its Psychological Correlates: A Meta-Analysis," *International Journal of Eating Disorders* 54, no. 7 (July 2021): 1073–1098, https://doi.org/10.1002/eat.23509.

12 Adapted from Evelyn Tribole and Elyse Resch, *Intuitive Eating: A Revolutionary Program That Works* (St. Martin's Griffin, 2003).

PART 1: MIDLIFE MAYHEM

1 N. Coslov, M. K. Richardson, and N. F. Woods, "'Not Feeling Like Myself' in Perimenopause—What Does It Mean? Observations from the Women Living Better Survey," *Menopause* 31, no. 5 (May 2024): 390–398, https://doi.org/10.1097/GME.0000000000002339.

2 R. Aljumah, S. Phillips, and J. C. Harper, "An Online Survey of Postmenopausal Women to Determine Their Attitudes and Knowledge of the Menopause," *Post Reproductive Health* 29, no. 2 (2023): 67–84, https://doi.org/10.1177/20533691231166543.

3 "Global Awareness Chasm About Menopause, First in Kind Research Reveals," Avon, July 28, 2020, https://www.avonworldwide.com/news/first-of-its-kind-research-on-menopause.

4 K. E. Reed, J. Camargo, J. Hamilton-Reeves, M. Kurzer, and M. Messina, "Neither Soy Nor Isoflavone Intake Affects Male T Reproductive Hormones: An Expanded and Updated Meta-Analysis of Clinical Studies," *Reproductive Toxicology* 100 (March 2021): 60–67, https://doi.org/10.1016/j.reprotox.2020.12.019.

5 "Perimenopause," CEMCOR, accessed December 19, 2024, https://www.cemcor.ca/resources/life-phases/perimenopause.

6 "State of Menopause Survey," Bonafide, https://hellobonafide.com/pages/state-of-menopause.

7 Y. Yang, U. A. Valdimarsdóttir, J. E. Manson, L. L. Sievert, B. L. Harlow, A. H. Eliassen, et al., "Premenstrual Disorders, Timing of Menopause, and Severity of Vasomotor Symptoms," *JAMA Network Open* 6, no. 9 (September 2023): e2334545, https://doi.org/10.1001/jamanetworkopen.2023.34545.

PART 2: WHAT TO EXPECT WHEN YOU'RE NOT EXPECTING PERIMENOPAUSE

1 J. S. Carpenter, Y. Sheng, C. D. Elomba, J. S. Alwine, M. Yue, C. A. Pike, et al., "A Systematic Review of Palpitations Prevalence by Menopausal Status," *Current Obstetrics Gynecology Reports* 10 (2021): 7–13, https://doi.org/10.1007/s13669-020-00302-z.

2 S. D. Harlow, S. A. M. Burnett-Bowie, G. A. Greendale, N. E. Avis, A. N. Reeves, T. R. Richards, et al., "Disparities in Reproductive Aging and Midlife Health Between Black and White Women: The Study of Women's Health Across the Nation (SWAN)," *Women's Midlife Health* 8, no. 3 (2022), https://doi.org/10.1186/s40695-022-00073-y.

3 A. L. Murkies, C. Lombard, B. J. Strauss, G. Wilcox, H. G. Burger, and M. S. Morton, "Dietary Flour Supplementation Decreases Post-Menopausal Hot Flushes: Effect of Soy and Wheat," *Maturitas* 21, no. 3 (April 1995): 189–195, https://doi.org/10.1016/0378-5122(95)00899-v.

4 M. N. Chen, C. C. Lin, and C. F. Liu, "Efficacy of Phytoestrogens for Menopausal Symptoms: A Meta-Analysis and Systematic Review," *Climacteric* 18, no. 2 (April 2015): 260–269, https://doi.org/10.3109/13697137.2014.966241; O. H. Franco, R. Chowdhury, J. Troup, T. Voortman, S. Kunutsor, M. Kavousi, et al., "Use of Plant-Based Therapies and Menopausal Symptoms: A Systematic Review and Meta-Analysis," *JAMA* 315, no. 23 (June 2016): 2554–2563, https://doi.org/10.1001/jama.2016.8012.

5 N. D. Barnard, H. Kahleova, D. N. Holtz, F. Del Aguila, M. Neola, L. M. Crosby, et al., "The Women's Study for the Alleviation of Vasomotor Symptoms (WAVS): A Randomized, Controlled Trial of a Plant-Based Diet and Whole Soybeans for Postmenopausal Women," *Menopause* 28, no. 10 (July 2021): 1150–1156, https://doi.org/10.1097/GME.0000000000001812; O. N. Furlong, H. J. Parr, S. J. Hodge, M. M. Slevin, E. E. Simpson, E. M. McSorley, et al., "Consumption of a Soy Drink Has No Effect on Cognitive Function but May Alleviate Vasomotor Symptoms in Post-Menopausal Women: A Randomised Trial," *European Journal of Nutrition* 59, no. 2 (March 2020): 755–766, https://doi.org/10.1007/s00394-019-01942-5.

6 G. C. Herber-Gast and G. D. Mishra, "Fruit, Mediterranean-Style, and High-Fat and -Sugar Diets Are Associated with the Risk of Night Sweats and Hot Flushes in Midlife: Results from a Prospective Cohort Study," *American Journal of Clinical Nutrition* 97, no. 5 (2013): 1092–1099, https://doi.org/10.3945/ajcn.112.049965.

7 C. Vetrani, L. Barrea, R. Rispoli, L. Verde, G. De Alteriis, A. Docimo, et al., "Mediterranean Diet: What Are the Consequences for Menopause?," *Front Endocrinol (Lausanne)* 25, no. 13 (2022): 886824, https://doi.org/10.3389/fendo.2022.886824.

8 G. Pounis, A. Di Castelnuovo, M. Bonaccio, S. Costanzo, M. Persichillo, V. Krogh, et al., "Flavonoid and Lignan Intake in a Mediterranean Population: Proposal for a Holistic Approach in Polyphenol Dietary Analysis, the Moli-Sani Study," *European Journal of Clinical Nutrition* 70, no. 3 (March 2016): 338–345, https://doi.org/10.1038/ejcn.2015.178.

9 2023 Nonhormone Therapy Position Statement Advisory Panel, "The 2023 Nonhormone Therapy Position Statement of the North American Menopause Society," *Menopause* 30, no. 6 (June 2023): 573–590, https://doi.org/10.1097/GME.0000000000002200.

10 D. Zhu, H. F. Chung, A. J. Dobson, N. Pandeya, D. J. Anderson, D. Kuh, et al., "Vasomotor Menopausal Symptoms and Risk of Cardiovascular Disease: A Pooled Analysis of Six Prospective Studies," *American Journal of Obstetrics & Gynecology* 223, no. 6 (December 2020): 898.e1-898.e16, https://doi.org/10.1016/j.ajog.2020.06.039.

11 M. de Zambotti , I. M. Colrain, H. S. Javitz, and F. C. Baker, "Magnitude of the Impact of Hot Flashes on Sleep in Perimenopausal Women," *Fertility and Sterility* 102, no. 6 (2014): 1708–1715.e1, https://doi.org/10.1016/j.fertnstert.2014.08.016.

12 P. Polo-Kantola, "Sleep Problems in Midlife and Beyond," *Maturitas* 68, no. 3 (2011): 224–232, https://doi.org/10.1016/j.maturitas.2010.12.009.

13 Y. Cui, K. Niu, C. Huang, H. Momma, L. Guan, Y. Kobayashi, et al., "Relationship Between Daily Isoflavone Intake and Sleep in Japanese Adults: A Cross-Sectional Study," *Nutrition Journal* 14, no. 127 (December 2015), https://doi.org/10.1186/s12937-015-0117-x.

14 E. Scoditti, M. R. Tumolo, and S. Garbarino, "Mediterranean Diet on Sleep: A Health Alliance," *Nutrients* 14, no. 14 (July 2022): 2998, https://doi.org/10.3390/nu14142998.

15 Y. Komada, I. Okajima, and T. Kuwata, "The Effects of Milk and Dairy Products on Sleep: A Systematic Review," *International Journal of Environmental Research and Public Health* 17, no. 24 (December 2020): 9440, https://doi.org/10.3390/ijerph17249440.

16 S. Mohsenian, S. Shabbidar, F. Siassi, M. Qorbani, S. Khosravi, M. Abshirini, et al., "Carbohydrate Quality Index: Its Relationship to Menopausal Symptoms in Postmenopausal Women," *Maturitas* 150 (August 2021): 42–48, https://doi.org/10.1016/j.maturitas.2021.05.006.

17 J. E. Gangwisch, L. Hale, M. P. St-Onge, L. Choi, E. S. LeBlanc, D. Malaspina, et al., "High Glycemic Index and Glycemic Load Diets as Risk Factors for Insomnia: Analyses from the Women's Health Initiative," *American Journal of Clinical Nutrition* 111, no. 2 (February 2020): 429–439, https://doi.org/10.1093/ajcn/nqz275.

18 A. Afaghi, H. O'Connor, and C. M. Chow, "High-Glycemic-Index Carbohydrate Meals Shorten Sleep Onset," *American Journal of Clinical Nutrition* 85, no. 2 (February 2007): 426–430, https://doi.org/10.1093/ajcn/85.2.426.

19 V. M. Hazzard, C. B. Burnette, L. Hooper, N. Larson, M. E. Eisenberg, and D. Neumark-Sztainer, "Lifestyle Health Behavior Correlates of Intuitive Eating in a Population-Based Sample of Men and Women," *Eating Behaviors* 46 (August 2022): 101644, https://doi.org/10.1016/j.eatbeh.2022.101644.

20 F. Auld, E. L. Maschauer, I. Morrison, D. Skene, and R. Riha, "Evidence for the Efficacy of Melatonin in the Treatment of Primary Adult Sleep Disorders," *Sleep Medicine Reviews* 34 (2017): 10–22, https://doi.org/10.1016/j.smrv.2016.06.005.

21 K. A. Guthrie, J. C. Larson, K. E. Ensrud, G. L. Anderson, J. S. Carpenter, E. W. Freeman, et al., "Effects of Pharmacologic and Nonpharmacologic Interventions on Insomnia Symptoms and Self-Reported Sleep Quality in Women with Hot Flashes: A Pooled Analysis of Individual Participant Data from Four MsFLASH Trials," *Sleep* 41, no. 1 (January 2018): zsx190, https://doi.org/10.1093/sleep/zsx190.

22 M. Sejbuk, I Mirończuk-Chodakowska, and A. M. Witkowska, "Sleep Quality: A Narrative Review on Nutrition, Stimulants, and Physical Activity as Important Factors," *Nutrients* 14, no. 9 (May 2022): 1912. https://doi.org/10.3390/nu14091912.

23 S. I. Iao, E. Jansen, K. Shedden , L. M. O'Brien, R. D. Chevrin, Kristin L. Knutson, et al., "Associations Between Bedtime Eating or Drinking, Sleep Duration and Wake After Sleep Onset: Findings from the American Time Use Survey," *British Journal of Nutrition* 127, no. 12 (2022): 1888–1897, https://doi.org/10.1017/S0007114521003597.

24 M. Zhao, M. Sun, R. Zhao, P. Chen, and S. Li, "Effects of Exercise on Sleep in Perimenopausal Women: A Meta-Analysis of Randomized Controlled Trials," *Explore (NY)* 19, no. 5 (September/October 2023): 636–645, https://doi.org/10.1016/j.explore.2023.02.001.

25 A. Arab, N. Rafie, R. Amani, and F. Shirani, "The Role of Magnesium in Sleep Health: A Systematic Review of Available Literature," *Biological Trace Element Research* 201, no. 1 (January 2023): 121–128, https://doi.org/10.1007/s12011-022-03162-1.

26 K. Barber and A. Charles, "Barriers to Accessing Effective Treatment and Support for Menopausal Symptoms: A Qualitative Study Capturing the Behaviours, Beliefs and Experiences of Key Stakeholders," *Patient Prefer Adherence* 2023, no. 17 (November 2023): 2971–2980, https://doi.org/10.2147/PPA.S430203.

27 A. Cano, S. Marshall, I. Zolfaroli, J. Bitzer, J. Ceausu, P. Chedraui, et al., "The Mediterranean Diet and Menopausal Health: An EMAS Position Statement," *Maturitas* 139 (Septemeber 2020): 90–97, https://doi.org/10.1016/j.maturitas.2020.07.001.

28 F. N. Jacka, A. O'Neil, R. Opie, C. Itsiopoulos, S. Cotton, M. Mohebbi, et al., "A Randomised Controlled Trial of Dietary Improvement for Adults with Major Depression (The 'Smiles' Trial)," *BMC Medicine* 15, no. 1 (January 2017): 23, https://doi.org/10.1186/s12916-017-0791-y.

29 S. J. Torres and C. A. Nowson, "A Moderate-Sodium DASH-Type Diet Improves Mood in Postmenopausal Women," *Nutrition* 28, no. 9 (September 2012): 896–900, https://doi.org/10.1016/j.nut.2011.11.029.

30 A. Hirose, M. Terauchi, M. Akiyoshi, Y. Owa, K. Kato, and T. Kubota, "Low-Dose Isoflavone Aglycone Alleviates Psychological Symptoms of Menopause in Japanese Women: A Randomized, Double-Blind, Placebo-Controlled Study," *Archives of Gynecology and Obstetrics* 293, no. 3 (March 2016): 609–15, https://doi.org/10.1007/s00404-015-3849-0.

31 J. Linardon, T. L. Tylka, and M. Fuller-Tyszkiewicz, "Intuitive Eating and Its Psychological Correlates: A Meta-Analysis," *International Journal of Eating Disorders* 54, no. 7 (July 2021): 1073–1098, https://doi.org/10.1002/eat.23509.

32 Z. Mei, O. Y. Addo, M. E. Jefferds, A. J. Sharma, R. C. Flores-Ayala, and G. M. Brittenham, "Physiologically Based Serum Ferritin Thresholds for Iron Deficiency in Children and Non-Pregnant Women: A US National Health and Nutrition Examination Surveys (NHANES) Serial Cross-Sectional Study," *Lancet Haematology* 8, no. 8 (August 2021): e572–e582, https://doi.org/10.1016/S2352-3026(21)00168-X.

33 C. Castelo-Branco and L. Quintas, "Iron Deficiency Without Anemia: Indications for Treatment," *Gynecological and Reproductive Endocrinology & Metabolism* 1, no. 4/2020 (November 2020): 215–222, https://doi.org/10.53260/GREM.201043.

34 R. M. J. Snipe, B. Brelis, Christina Kappas, J. K. Young, L. Eishold, J. M. Chui, et al., "Omega-3 Long Chain Polyunsaturated Fatty Acids as a Potential Treatment for Reducing Dysmenorrhoea Pain: Systematic Literature Review and Meta-Analysis," *Nutrition & Dietetics* 81, no. 1 (February 2024): 94–106, https://doi.org/10.1111/1747-0080.12835.

35 F. Abdi, M. A. Amjadi, F. Zaheri, and F. A. Rahnemaei, "Role of Vitamin D and Calcium in the Relief of Primary Dysmenorrhea: A Systematic Review," *Obstetrics & Gynecology Science* 64, no. 1 (January 2021): 13–26, https://doi.org/10.5468/ogs.20205.

36 S. Zarei, S. Mohammad-Alizadeh-Charandabi, M. Mirghafourvand, Y. Javadzadeh, and F. Effati-Daryani, "Effects of Calcium-Vitamin D and Calcium-Alone on Pain Intensity and Menstrual Blood Loss in Women with Primary Dysmenorrhea: A Randomized Controlled Trial," *Pain Medicine* 18, no. 1 (January 2017): 3–13, https://doi.org/10.1093/pm/pnw121.

37 K.-C. Lin, K.-J. Huang, M.-N. Lin, C.-Y. Wang, and T.-Y. Tsai, "Vitamin D Supplementation for Patients with Dysmenorrhoea: A Meta-Analysis with Trial Sequential Analysis of Randomised Controlled Trials," *Nutrients* 16, no. 7 (April 2024): 1089, https://doi.org/10.3390/nu16071089. PMID: 38613122; PMCID: PMC11013696.

38 M. Armour, C. C. Ee, D. Naidoo, Z. Ayati, K. J. Chalmers, K. A. Steel, et al., "Exercise for Dysmenorrhoea," *Cochrane Database of Systematic Reviews* 9 (2019): 1465–1858, https://doi.org/10.1002/14651858.CD004142.pub4.

39 E. Volpi, R, Nazemi, and S. Fujita, "Muscle Tissue Changes with Aging," *Current Opinion in Clinical Nutrition and Metabolic Care* 7, no. 4 (July 2004): 405–410, https://doi.org/10.1097/01.mco.0000134362.76653.b2. PMID: 15192443; PMCID: PMC2804956.

40 A. I. Sánchez-Rosales, A. L. Guadarrama-López, L. S. Gaona-Valle, B. E. Martínez-Carrillo, and R. Valdés-Ramos, "The Effect of Dietary Patterns on Inflammatory Biomarkers in Adults with Type 2 Diabetes Mellitus: A Systematic Review and Meta-Analysis of Randomized Controlled Trials," *Nutrients* 14, no. 21 (October 2022): 4577, https://doi.org/10.3390/nu14214577.

41 Z. Tajary, Z. Esmaeily, M. Rezaei, S. Daei, A. Eyvazkhani, M. M. Dara, et al., "Musculoskeletal Pain Is Associated with Dietary Diversity Score among Community-Dwelling Older Adult: A Cross-Sectional Study," *International Journal of Food Science* (February 2022), https://doi.org/10.1155/2022/4228925.

42 J. Bajerska, K. Łagowska, M. Mori, J. Regula, A. Skoczek-Rubińska, T. Toda, et al., "A Meta-Analysis of Randomized Controlled Trials of the Effects of Soy Intake on Inflammatory Markers in Postmenopausal Women," *Journal of Nutrition* 152, no. 1 (January 2022): 5–15, https://doi.org/10.1093/jn/nxab325.

43 K. Prokopidis, M. Mazidi, R. Sankaranarayanan, B. Tajik, A. McArdle, and M. Isanejad, "Effects of Whey and Soy Protein Supplementation on Inflammatory Cytokines in Older Adults: A Systematic Review and Meta-Analysis," *British Journal of Nutrition* 129, no. 5 (March 2023): 759–770, https://doi.org/10.1017/S0007114522001787.

44 M. N. Turner, D. O. Hernandez, W. Cade, C. P. Emerson, J. M. Reynolds, and T. M. Best, "The Role of Resistance Training Dosing on Pain and Physical Function in Individuals with Knee Osteoarthritis: A Systematic Review," *Sports Health* 12, no. 2 (March/April 2020): 200–206, https://doi.org/10.1177/1941738119887183.

45 G. A. Greendale, M.-H. Huang, R. G. Wight, T. Seeman, C. Luetters, N. E. Avis, et al., "Effects of the Menopause Transition and Hormone Use on Cognitive Performance in Midlife Women," *Neurology* 72, no. 21 (May 26, 2009): 1850–1857, https://doi.org/10.1212/WNL.0b013e3181a71193. PMID: 19470968; PMCID: PMC2690984.

46 L. Mosconi, V. Berti, J. Dyke, E. Schelbaum, S. Jett, L. Loughlin, et al., "Menopause Impacts Human Brain Structure, Connectivity, Energy Metabolism, and Amyloid-Beta Deposition," *Scientific Reports* 11, no. 1 (June 2021): 10867, https://doi.org/10.1038/s41598-021-90084-y.

47 G. A. Greendale, A. S. Karlamangla, and P. M. Maki, "The Menopause Transition and Cognition," *JAMA* 323, no. 15 (April 2020): 1495–1496, https://doi.org/10.1001/jama.2020.1757.

48 J. Skrynka and B. T. Vincent, "Hunger Increases Delay Discounting of Food and Non-Food Rewards," *Psychonomic Bulletin & Review* 26, no. 5 (October 2019): 1729–1737, https://doi.org/10.3758/s13423-019-01655-0.

49 J. Fu, L. J. Tan, J. E. Lee, and S. Shin, "Association Between the Mediterranean Diet and Cognitive Health Among Healthy Adults: A Systematic Review and Meta-Analysis," *Frontiers in Nutrition* 28, no. 9 (July 2022): 946361, https://doi.org/10.3389/fnut.2022.946361.

50 A. Tessier , M. Cortese, C. Yuan, K. Bjornevik, A. Ascherio, D. Wang, et al., "Consumption of Olive Oil and Diet Quality and Risk of Dementia-Related Death," *JAMA* 7, no. 5 (May 2024): e2410021, https://doi.org/10.1001/jamanetworkopen.2024.10021.

51 C. Marshall, C. Lengyel, and A. Utioh, "Body Dissatisfaction Among Middle-Aged and Older Women," *Canadian Journal of Dietetic Practice and Research* 73, no. 2 (2012): e241–e247, https://doi.org/10.3148/73.2.2012.e241.

52 E. Cameron, P. Ward, S. A. Mandville-Anstey, and A. Coombs, "The Female Aging Body: A Systematic Review of Female Perspectives on Aging, Health, and Body Image," *Journal of Women & Aging* 31, no. 1 (January/February 2019): 3–17, https://doi.org/10.1080/08952841.2018.1449586.

53 P. Jacquet, Y. Schutz, J. P. Montani, and A. Dulloo, "How Dieting Might Make Some Fatter: Modeling Weight Cycling Toward Obesity from a Perspective of Body Composition Autoregulation," *International Journal of Obesity* 44, no. 6 (June 2020): 1243–1253, https://doi.org/10.1038/s41366-020-0547-1.

54 G. James, "The Average Woman Has Been on 61 Diets by Age 45, Poll Reveals," HuffPost (May 20, 2012): https://www.huffingtonpost.co.uk/2012/03/20/average-woman-61-diets-age-45_n_1366665.

55 C. B. Martin, K. A. Herrick, N. Sarafrazi, and C. L. Ogden, "Attempts to Lose Weight Among Adults in the United States," CDC, July 2018: https://www.cdc.gov/nchs/products/databriefs/db313.htm.

56 Naomi Wolf, Chapter 6, "Hunger," in *The Beauty Myth: How Images of Beauty Are Used Against Women* (Chatto & Windus, 1990), 187.

57 A. Moilanen, J. Kopra, H. Kröger, R. Sund, T. Rikkonen, and J. Sirola, "Characteristics of Long-Term Femoral Neck Bone Loss in Postmenopausal Women: A 25-Year Follow-Up," *Journal of Bone and Mineral Research* 37, no. 2 (February 2022): 173–178, https://doi.org/10.1002/jbmr.4444.

58 M. M. Nowak, M. Niemczyk, S. Gołębiewski, and L. Pączek, "Impact of Body Mass Index on All-Cause Mortality in Adults: A Systematic Review and Meta-Analysis," *Journal of Clinical Medicine* 13, no. 8 (April 2024): 2305, https://doi.org/10.3390/jcm13082305.

59 E. M. Matheson, D. E. King, and C. J. Everett, "Healthy Lifestyle Habits and Mortality in Overweight and Obese Individuals," *American Board of Family Medicine* 25, no. 1 (January/February 2012): 9–15, 10.3122/jabfm.2012.01.110164.

60 I. Carrard, S. Rothen, and R. F. Rodgers, "Body Image Concerns and Intuitive Eating in Older Women," *Appetite* 164 (September 2021): 105275, https://doi.org/10.1016/j.appet.2021.105275.

61 L. S. Kilpela , S. C. Hooper, C. L. Strand, V. B. Marshall, C. L. Verzijl, T. M. Stewart, et al., "The Longitudinal Associations of Body Dissatisfaction with Health and Wellness Behaviors in Midlife and Older Women," *International Journal of Environmental Research and Public Health* 20, no. 24 (December 2023): 7143, https://doi.org/10.3390/ijerph20247143.

62 R. E. Nappi and M. Kokot-Kierepa, "Vaginal Health: Insights, Views & Attitudes (VIVA)—Results from an International Survey," *Climacteric* 15, no. 1 (February 2012): 36–44, https://doi.org/10.3109/13697137.2011.647840.

63 E. Moyneur, K. Dea, L. R. Derogatis, F. Vekeman, A. Y. Dury, and F. Labrie, "Prevalence of Depression and Anxiety in Women Newly Diagnosed with Vulvovaginal Atrophy and Dyspareunia," *Menopause* 27, no. 2 (February 2020): 134–142, https://doi.org/10.1097/GME.0000000000001450.

64 "About Women and Heart Disease," CDC, May 15, 2024, https://www.cdc.gov/heart-disease/about/women-and-heart-disease.html.

65 S.A. Peters and M. Woodward, "Women's Reproductive Factors and Incident Cardiovascular Disease in the UK Biobank," *Heart* 104, no. 13 (July 2018): 1069–1075, https://doi.org/10.1136/heartjnl-2017-312289.

66 J. S. Brand, Y. T. van der Schouw, N. C. Onland-Moret, S. J. Sharp, K. K. Ong, K.-T. Khaw, et al., "Age at Menopause, Reproductive Life Span, and Type 2 Diabetes Risk: Results from the Epic-Interact Study," *Diabetes Care* 36, no. 4 (April 2013): 1012–1019, https://doi.org/10.2337/dc12-1020.

67 H.-F. Chung, A. J. Dobson, K. Hayashi, R. Hardy, D. Kuh, D. J. Anderson, et al., "Ethnic Differences in the Association Between Age at Natural Menopause and Risk of Type 2 Diabetes Among Postmenopausal Women: A Pooled Analysis of Individual Data From 13 Cohort Studies," *Diabetes Care* 46, no. 11 (November 2023): 2024–2034, https://doi.org/10.2337/dc23-1209.

68 F. Hosseini, A. Jayedi, T. A. Khan, and S. Shab-Bidar, "Dietary Carbohydrate and the Risk of Type 2 Diabetes: An Updated Systematic Review and Dose-Response Meta-Analysis of Prospective Cohort Studies," *Scientific Reports* 12, no. 1 (February 2022): 2491, https://doi.org/10.1038/s41598-022-06212-9.

69 F. L. P. Soares, M. H. Ramos, M. Gramelisch, R. de Paula Pego Silva, J. da Silva Batista, M. Cattafesta, et al., "Intuitive Eating Is Associated with Glycemic Control in Type 2 Diabetes," *Eating and Weight Disorders* 26, no. 2 (March 2021): 599–608, https://doi.org/10.1007/s40519-020-00894-8.

70 L. DiPietro, A. Gribok, M. S. Stevens, L. F. Hamm, and W. Rumpler, "Three 15-Min Bouts of Moderate Postmeal Walking Significantly Improves 24-H Glycemic Control in Older People at Risk for Impaired Glucose Tolerance," *Diabetes Care* 36, no. 10 (October 2013): 3262–3268, https://doi.org/10.2337/dc13-0084.

71 S. M. Nachvak, S. Moradi, J. Anjom-Shoae, J. Rahmani, M. Nasiri, V. Maleki, et al., "Soy, Soy Isoflavones, and Protein Intake in Relation to Mortality from All Causes, Cancers, and Cardiovascular Diseases: A Systematic Review and Dose-Response Meta-Analysis of Prospective Cohort Studies," *Journal of the Academy of Nutrition and Dietetics* 119, no. 9 (September 2019): 1483–1500.e17, https://doi.org/10.1016/j.jand.2019.04.011.

72 J. Qi, R. Zhu, J. Mao, X. Wang, H. Xu, and L. Guo, "Effect of Unfermented Soy Product Consumption on Blood Lipids in Postmenopausal Women: A Systematic Review and Meta-Analysis of Randomized Controlled Trials," *Journal of the Academy of Nutrition and Dietetics* 124, no. 11 (November 2024): 1474–1491.e1, https://doi.org/10.1016/j.jand.2024.02.006.

73 P. Surampudi, B. Enkhmaa, E. Anuurad, and L. Berglund, "Lipid Lowering with Soluble Dietary Fiber," *Current Atherosclerosis Reports* 18, no. 12 (December 2016): 75, https://doi.org/10.1007/s11883-016-0624-z. PMID: 27807734.

74 "Osteoporosis and Fractures," National Osteoporosis Foundation, April 2016, https://www.bonehealthandosteoporosis.org/wp-content/uploads/2016/04/Osteoporosis-and-Fractures.pdf.

75 A. S. Karlamangla, S. M. Burnett-Bowie, and C. J. Crandall, "Bone Health During the Menopause Transition and Beyond," *Obstetrics and Gynecology Clinics* 45, no. 4 (December 2018): 695–708, https://doi.org/10.1016/j.ogc.2018.07.012. Epub 2018 Oct 25. PMID: 30401551; PMCID: PMC6226267.

76 M. M. Shams-White, M. Chung, M. Du, Z. Fu, K. L. Insogna, M. C. Karlsen, et al., "Dietary Protein and Bone Health: A Systematic Review and Meta-Analysis from the National Osteoporosis Foundation," *American Journal of Clinical Nutrition* 105, no. 6 (June 2017): 1528–1543, https://doi.org/10.3945/ajcn.116.145110.

77 X. Zhang, X.-O. Shu, H. Li, G. Yang, Q. Li, Y. T. Gao, et al., "Prospective Cohort Study of Soy Food Consumption and Risk of Bone Fracture Among Postmenopausal Women," *Archives of Internal Medicine* 165, no. 16 (September 2005): 1890–1895, https://doi.org/10.1001/archinte.165.16.1890.

78 R. V. Seimon , A. L. Wild-Taylor, S. E. Keating, S. McClintock, C. Harper, A. A. Gibson, et al., "Effect of Weight Loss via Severe vs Moderate Energy Restriction on Lean Mass and Body Composition Among Postmenopausal Women with Obesity: The TEMPO Diet Randomized Clinical Trial," *JAMA* 2, no. 10 (2019): e1913733, https://doi.org/10.1001/jamanetworkopen.2019.13733.

PART 3: THE FOUNDATIONS OF A NOURISHED MENOPAUSE

1 J. W. Erdman Jr., "AHA Science Advisory: Soy Protein and Cardiovascular Disease: A Statement for Healthcare Professionals from the Nutrition Committee of the AHA," *Circulation* 102, no. 20 (November 2000): 2555-9, https://doi.org/10.1161/01.cir.102.20.2555. PMID: 11076833.

2 C. Cui , R. L. Birru, B. E. Snitz, M. Ihara, C. Kakuta, B. J. Lopresti, et al., "Effects of Soy Isoflavones on Cognitive Function: A Systematic Review and Meta-Analysis of Randomized Controlled Trials," *Nutrition Reviews* 78, no. 2 (February 2020): 134–144, https://doi.org/10.1093/nutrit/nuz050; J. P. D. Kleinloog, L. Tischmann, R. P. Mensink, T. C. Adam, and P. J. Joris, "Longer-Term Soy Nut Consumption Improves Cerebral Blood Flow and Psychomotor Speed: Results of a Randomized, Controlled Crossover Trial in Older Men and Women," *American Journal of Clinical Nutrition* 114, no. 6 (December 2021): 2097–2106, https://doi.org/10.1093/ajcn/nqab289.

3 Y. Hu, Y. Li, L. Sampson, M. Wang, J. E. Manson, E. Rimm, et al., "Lignan Intake and Risk of Coronary Heart Disease," *Journal of the American College of Cardiology* 78, no. 7 (August 2021): 666–678, https://doi.org/10.1016/j.jacc.2021.05.049.

4 J. Otun, A. Sahebkar, L. Östlundh, S. L. Atkin, and T. Sathyapalan, "Systematic Review and Meta-Analysis on the Effect of Soy on Thyroid Function," *Scientific Reports* 9, no. 1 (March 2019): 3964, https://doi.org/10.1038/s41598-019-40647-x.

5 J. Y. Dong and L. Q. Qin, "Soy Isoflavones Consumption and Risk of Breast Cancer Incidence or Recurrence: A Meta-Analysis of Prospective Studies," *Breast Cancer Research and Treatment* 125 (2011): 315–323, https://doi.org/10.1186/gm211.

6 S.-A. Lee, X.-O. Shu, H. Li , G. Yang, H. Cai, W. Wen, et al., "Adolescent and Adult Soy Food Intake and Breast Cancer Risk: Results from the Shanghai Women's Health Study," *American Journal of Clinical Nutrition* 89, no. 6 (June 2009): 1920–1926, https://doi.org/10.3945/ajcn.2008.27361.

7 F. F. Zhang, D. E. Haslam, M. B. Terry, J. A. Knight, I. L. Andrulis, M. B. Daly, et al., "Dietary Isoflavone Intake and All-Cause Mortality in Breast Cancer Survivors: The Breast Cancer Family Registry," *Cancer* 123, no. 11 (June 2017): 2070–2079, https://doi.org/10.1002/cncr.30615.

8 J. M. Beasley, A. Z. LaCroix, M. L. Neuhouser, Y. Huang, L. Tinker, N. Woods, et al., "Protein Intake and Incident Frailty in the Women's Health Initiative Observational Study," *Journal of the American Geriatrics Society* 58, no. 6 (June 2010): 1063–1071, https://doi.org/10.1111/j.1532-5415.2010.02866.x.

9 E. J. Arentson-Lantz, D. K. Layman, H. J. Leidy, W. W. Campbell, and S. M. Phillips, "Important Concepts in Protein Nutrition, Aging, and Skeletal Muscle: Honoring Dr. Douglas Paddon-Jones (1969–2021) by Highlighting His Research Contributions," *Journal of Nutrition* 153, no. 3 (March 2023): 615–621, https://doi.org/10.1016/j.tjnut.2023.01.011.

10 U.S. Department of Agriculture and the Agricultural Research Service, "What We Eat in America: Nutrient Intakes from Food by Gender and Age," *National Health and Nutrition Examination Survey (NHANES) 2009–10*, December 4, 2014, http://www.ars.usda.gov/Sp2 userfiles/Place/12355000/Pdf/0910/Table_1_Nin_Gen_09.Pdf.

11 A. Reynolds, J. Mann, J. Cummings, N. Winter, E. Mete, and L. Te Morenga, "Carbohydrate Quality and Human Health: A Series of Systematic Reviews and Meta-Analyses," *Lancet* 393, no. 10170 (February 2019): 434–445, https://doi.org/10.1016/S0140-6736(18)31809-9.

12 P. Surampudi, B. Enkhmaa, E. Anuurad, and L. Berglund, "Lipid Lowering with Soluble Dietary Fiber," *Current Atherosclerosis Reports* 18, no. 12 (December 2016): 75, https://doi.org/10.1007/s11883-016-0624-z.

13 S. Mohsenian, S. Shabbidar, F. Siassi, M. Qorbani, S. Khosravi, M. Abshirini, et al., "Carbohydrate Quality Index: Its Relationship to Menopausal Symptoms in Postmenopausal Women," *Maturitas* 150 (August 2021): 42–48, https://doi.org/10.1016/j.maturitas.2021.05.006.

14 D. Aune, D. S. Chan, R. Lau, R. Vieira, D. C. Greenwood, E. Kampman, et al., "Dietary Fibre, Whole Grains, and Risk of Colorectal Cancer: Systematic Review and Dose-Response Meta-Analysis of Prospective Studies," *BMJ* 343 (November 2011): d6617, https://doi.org/10.1136/bmj.d6617.

15 K. E. Charlton, L. C. Tapsell, M. J. Batterham, J. O'Shea, R. Thorne, E. Beck, et al., "Effect of 6 Weeks' Consumption of B-Glucan-Rich Oat Products on Cholesterol Levels in Mildly Hypercholesterolaemic Overweight Adults," *British Journal of Nutrition* 107, no. 7 (April 2012): 1037–1047, https://doi.org/10.1017/S0007114511003850.

16 D. D. Wang , Y. Li, S. N. Bhupathiraju, B. A. Rosner, Q. Sun, E. L. Giovannucci, et al., "Fruit and Vegetable Intake and Mortality: Results From 2 Prospective Cohort Studies of US Men and Women and a Meta-Analysis of 26 Cohort Studies," *Circulation* 143, no. 17 (April 2021): 1642–1654, https://doi.org/10.1161/CIRCULATIONAHA.120.048996.

17 Y. Komada, I. Okajima, and T. Kuwata, "The Effects of Milk and Dairy Products on Sleep: A Systematic Review," *International Journal of Environmental Research and Public Health* 17, no. 24 (December 2020): 9440, https://doi.org/10.3390/ijerph17249440.

18 L. C. Kahwati, R. P. Weber, H. Pan, M. Gourlay, E. LeBlanc, M. Coker-Schwimmer, et al. "Vitamin D, Calcium, or Combined Supplementation for the Primary Prevention of Fractures in Community-Dwelling Adults: Evidence Report and Systematic Review for the US Preventive Services Task Force," *JAMA* 319, no. 15 (April 2018): 1600–1612, https://doi.org/10.1001/jama.2017.21640.

19 "Calcium: Fact Sheet for Health Professional," *National Institutes of Health*, updated July 24, 2024, https://ods.od.nih.gov/factsheets/Calcium-Health Professional.

20 T.-C. Su, J.-J. Hwang, K.-C. Huang, F.-T. Chiang, K.-L. Chien, K.-Y. Wang, et al., "A Randomized, Double-Blind, Placebo-Controlled Clinical Trial to Assess the Efficacy and Safety of Ethyl-Ester Omega-3 Fatty Acid in Taiwanese Hypertriglyceridemic Patients," *Journal of Atherosclerosis and Thrombosis* 24, no. 3 (March 2017): 275–289, https://doi.org/10.5551/jat.34231.

21 X. Zhang, J. A. Ritonja, N. Zhou, B. E. Chen, and X. Li, "Omega-3 Polyunsaturated Fatty Acids Intake and Blood Pressure: A Dose-Response Meta-Analysis of Randomized Controlled Trials," *Journal of the American Heart Association* 11, no. 11 (June 2022): e025071, https://doi.org/10.1161/JAHA.121.025071.

22 B. M. Anderson and D. W. L. Ma, "Are All N-3 Polyunsaturated Fatty Acids Created Equal?," *Lipids in Health and Disease* 8 (August 2009): 33, https://doi.org/10.1186/1476-511X-8-33.

23 C. Franchi, I. Ardiono, C. Bosetti, E. Negri, D. Serraino, A. Crispo, et al., "Inverse Association between Canned Fish Consumption and Colorectal Cancer Risk: Analysis of Two Large Case-Control Studies," *Nutrients* 14, no. 8 (April 2022): 1663, https://doi.org/10.3390/nu14081663.

COOLING AND COMFORTING DRINKS

1 F. Idowu-Adebayo, V. Fogliano, and A. Linnemann, "Turmeric-Fortified Cow and Soya Milk: Golden Milk as a Street Food to Support Consumer Health," *Foods* 11, no. 4 (February 2022): 558, https://doi.org/10.3390/foods11040558.

RESOURCES

Books

Tribole, Evelyn, and Elyse Resch. *Intuitive Eating: A Revolutionary Anti-Diet Approach*. 4th ed. St. Martin's Essentials, 2020.

Harrison, Christy. *Anti-Diet: Reclaim Your Time, Money, Well-Being, and Happiness Through Intuitive Eating*. Little, Brown Spark, 2019.

Beckett, Emma. *You Are More Than What You Eat: Science, Nutrition, and a Perfectly Imperfect Approach to Eating*. Pantera Press, 2024.

Professional Organizations

The Menopause Society—https:// www.menopause.org

The International Menopause Society—https:// www.imsociety.org

The Canadian Menopause Society—https://www.canadianmenopausesociety.org

Intuitive Eating Professionals Directory—https://www. intuitiveeating.org

Online Health and Wellness Resources

The Midlife and Menopause Un-Dieters Guide to Intuitive Eating. Bonus self-paced course—https://www.menopausenutritionist.ca/bookresources

The Midlife Feast online community—https://www.menopausenutritionist.ca/themidlifefeastcommunity

Buff Bones Exercise for Osteoporosis—https://buff-bones.com

Yoga for Menopause, Niamh Daly—https://yinstinctyoga.com

CBTi for Insomnia—https://mysleepwell.ca

Dr. Maria Luque, Menopause Fitness—https://www.drmarialuque.com

Christine Chessman, Non-Diet Trainer—https://hellofitnesschristine.com

Menopause Symptom Tracking Tools—https://www.herstasis.com/menopause-diagnostic-tools

ACKNOWLEDGMENTS

Thank you for bringing this book into your kitchen and trusting me to be your guide.

One of my earliest memories is sneaking into the kitchen at dawn to make bread. In my mind, all you needed to make bread was flour, water, and love. I'd proudly present my creation to my parents, who, despite the early hour and crude concoction, always took a bite and proclaimed it delicious. Over the years, there would be many other concoctions created in that kitchen ranging from oyster sandwiches for parents while my friends and I performed gymnastics in the backyard to my dad's favorite comfort foods before he died.

My dad, our town's OB-GYN, was also my first boss. He gave me my first part-time job in his office. Even though I spent most of my time with a filing cabinet, I couldn't help but notice the experiences of the women he treated, especially when symptoms like hot flashes knocked them off their feet. I also remember the collective panic in 2002 when the Women's Health Initiative (WHI) study results were released, causing many to fear hormone therapy. I recall him asking me if I knew of any natural alternatives he could offer his patients, many of whom were too scared to stay on hormones.

So, it didn't surprise me when I developed a deep interest in women's health and nutrition or that my love of making nourishing food would inspire me to manage my own early menopause with nutrition, because food is my love language and always has been.

I became a dietitian and naturopathic doctor because I believed in the power of food to help nourish and take care of us and those we love. It wasn't until I become a certified intuitive eating counselor that I appreciated how important it was to have a flexible and forgiving relationship with food, especially in midlife and menopause.

Many of these recipes were written for my patients when they needed quick and easy meals to help them manage some of the symptoms they were experiencing in perimenopause and menopause. But, when I found myself in early perimenopause at thirty-seven, they also became part of my story. I hope these recipes bring comfort and ease to your midlife journey as well.

To Brent, Maeve, Maren, and Beckett: Thank you for letting this book take over our lives (often too much!) and cheering me on every step of the way. You are my reason for everything, and I love you all so much for believing in me. And to my mom, Betty, thank you for telling me I could do anything from the moment I was born and for reminding me at the exact times I needed to hear it.

To my sister Friedel, thank you for being the best sister, friend, and recipe tester I could ever ask for. I promise to keep you well fed in our Golden Girls house.

To my friends and colleagues who generously lent their time and encouragement—thank you. Your support and insights were invaluable, and I am deeply grateful.

To the dream team of photographer Alexandra Grablewski and stylist Cyd McDowell, thank you for bringing my vision of the recipes to life on these pages. Your skills and expertise made it so easy to trust the process and know that everything would turn out beautifully.

To my editors, Judy Pray and Kylie Foxx McDonald, and the team at Workman Publishing, I can't thank you enough for patiently holding this first-time author's hand through every step of this process. I feel so lucky to have landed in your capable hands and know that this book is better because of it.

This cookbook would not exist without the help of my agent, Katherine Cowles. Thank you for helping me bring my dream to life. I'll be forever grateful that you took a chance on me.

To the community of Feasters who continue to inspire me, thank you. Your stories are part of this cookbook and will bring comfort and hope to others who are feeling lost in the storm of menopause.

INDEX

Page references in *italics* indicate photographs.

C

D

E

F

S

T

U

V

W

Y

Z

ABOUT THE AUTHOR

Dr. Jenn Salib Huber, RD, ND, is a Canadian Registered Dietitian, Naturopathic Doctor, and Certified Intuitive Eating Counselor with more than twenty years of experience helping women navigate the physical and emotional changes of perimenopause and menopause. With a unique blend of expertise in nutrition, integrative medicine, and intuitive eating, she's on a mission to help women experience food as a source of joy, connection, and nourishment, in all seasons of life.

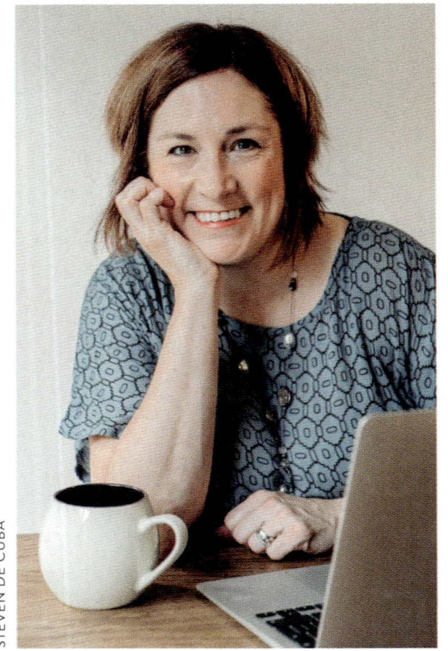

STEVEN DE CUBA

Dr. Jenn is the host of *The Midlife Feast* podcast and online community, where she offers practical tools and compassionate support to women who want to learn how to manage menopause without diets and food rules.

A proud Canadian, Dr. Jenn currently lives in Europe with her husband, children, and cats.